Keith Laun

Getting Better:

My Journey through Transverse Myelitis and Lessons for Health Care Professionals, Patients and Families

This book is dedicated to the thousands of health care professionals who truly care about their jobs, their patients and their institutions, and who insist on making a positive difference every day.

We thank you!

Table of Contents

Introduction

What you are about to read is all true. The names (all but ours) have been changed and we have deliberately not mentioned the names of any of the hospitals we had any involvement with. It doesn't matter; the nurses and doctors could be any nurses and doctors, and the hospitals could be any hospitals. We, on the other hand, are just two fairly ordinary people who had this bizarre experience from which we grew both in terms of our faith and in our knowledge about America's health care system. Our story contains elements of journey, of faith, of humor, of sarcasm (sorry in advance to those of you who don't appreciate sarcasm as humor) and lessons learned which we wanted to share with those who can make changes in how our health system works and with those who may be patients or the advocates of patients in the system.

Our outcome is positive, at least so far, so there is no unhappy ending to fear but our hope is that this tale of our journey through this strange and difficult time will enrich your lives in some way. It may be as doctors and nurses, it may be as patients, it may be as caregivers, bureaucrats, spiritual people, patients in hospitals, or a business student looking for a case study through which to examine health care; whoever you are, we wish you well!

"Sometimes something happens that is so catastrophic it is impossible for a while – or even for a long time – to see beyond the darkness, even to believe that there *is* anything beyond it. But there always is." Mary Balogh "At Last Comes Love"

Chapter 1 - Spinal Shock

My annual visit to my doctor, Paul Lawrence, in April of 2010 was fun as usual, or at least as fun as a visit to the doctor can be! I really enjoyed talking with Paul, he shares my quirky sense of humor, and this year there wasn't much of a medical nature to discuss. He couldn't fault me for my lifestyle; I didn't smoke, I wasn't overweight, I drank an occasional glass of wine, and I exercised on a regular basis. I was happy at home, I loved my wife, I adored our grandchildren, and I was not stressed at work. I had previously had some mysterious fainting spells, which after a good deal of testing had finally been diagnosed two years prior as atonic seizures (these are misrouted electrical charges in the brain that do not result in the spasms normally associated with the word "seizure") and as long as I took my daily doses of medication, I had no trouble at all.

The results of my blood tests were normal, and this worried me the way that some things do when they sound too good to be true, like when the kids are too quiet or when a company sends you something telling you (and all your neighbors) that "you are a lucky winner in a sweepstake". I don't think I had ever had a completely perfect blood test before; usually there was *something* to be concerned about, cholesterol, triglycerides, etc., but this time everything was in order, and I was apparently a fine specimen of health.

On July 19th I asked Wendy (our pet name for our Wii Fit) to tell me what my physical age was, and she told me 33. This was a full 25 years off my real age but 19 more than the number of birthdays I had celebrated (thanks to Julius Caesar who invented my birthday to fix the calendar every four years). Actually I wanted to agree with Wendy, I felt I was in the best shape of my life, and I had never felt better! Everything was terrific!

Day 1

The very next day, on July 20th, 2010, my wife (Claire) and I were upgraded on an uneventful flight (the very BEST kind) from Boston to San Francisco to teach a three day class. Upon arrival I was walking towards baggage claim when I was suddenly struck by this incredible pain in my rib cage. Claire asked me how severe it was, on a scale of 1 being hardly noticeable, to 10 being the most severe pain I could imagine, and I told her it was an 8! She asked me all kinds of questions: where exactly was it? When did it start? Was it sharp? Dull? Aching? What else could I tell her to describe it? Neither of us had any idea what it was, although like most people, we speculated.

It could be gall bladder, appendicitis, a kidney stone, or even food poisoning! Neither of us had ever experienced any pain like it, so we had nothing to compare it to. Claire told me to go sit down while she got the bags, and we would see how I felt then. I sat down on a chair in the baggage claim area while Claire collected the suitcases, and when I told her the pain had not relented, she told me to take a taxi directly to the hospital. She, on the other hand, would take the suitcases to our hotel, check in, and then take another taxi and meet me at the Emergency Room. I painfully walked downstairs, waited in the taxi line for about ten minutes, and took a taxi to the local hospital.

I arrived at the Emergency Room and was seen right away (just say "pain in my chest" and it clears the way for all kinds of medical assistance!) The doctor (Dr. Ryan) asked me to describe my pain and when I told him it was in my chest he immediately started looking for a heart problem, but that was quickly ruled out by an EKG. He had no idea what was causing the pain, but he had a solution!

He gave me a powerful painkiller, Dilaudid. This drug immediately made me nauseous (a known side effect of many pain medications) and I vomited profusely. Then he scheduled me for a Chest X ray, had a nurse (Jeanne) take some blood for testing, and asked me for a urine sample. For the first time in my life I was incapable of urinating! Until I could produce some, I just lay there.

I was still in intense pain, still not urinating, and groggy from all the drugs they had been giving me when our ER nurse, Jeanne, came into our cubicle with another nurse, whom she introduced as Lee. She told us that Lee would be the nurse who would be responsible for our care for the next twelve hours, or, until we left. Jeanne explained to Lee, right in front of us, what my status was, what had been done so far, and what they were waiting for (which in this case was the urine sample) and as a result Lee knew everything about my history and status, and we knew everything that they knew! It was very reassuring that there were no secrets, nothing hidden, and no plans that we weren't a part of. It was one of the most helpful things during the entire experience!

In the end, it took me 5 hours before I was able to produce any urine, and then it was very little. The lab ran the tests and Dr. Ryan was able to rule out kidney stones, gall bladder problems, appendicitis, spleen, liver and any other organ malfunction. He then decided to do a CT scan for which I had to drink a solution (they called it contrast and said it would help "enhance the image").

11

Unfortunately that also made me nauseous, and after I vomited a few more times someone took me to have my CT scan. Then the doctor reported that he couldn't find anything wrong, except that it appeared that I had a lot of stool in my intestine. So the new nurse gave me a bottle of magnesium citrate which she assured me would solve the problem, but she told me that I could always come back if things didn't get any better.

Claire called for a taxi, and on the ride back to our hotel from the hospital I impressed the driver by my ability to vomit on three separate occasions, twice because of the drugs I had been given, and once I think was because of his driving. He must have prepared for his driving test by watching "fast and furious" because he seemed to be in some kind of race, but it might just have been his desire to get me out of his cab! We finally arrived at the hotel and went straight up to our room where I drank the magnesium citrate which tasted revolting and went to bed, hoping for the promised relief overnight, and praying for a rapid recovery!

Day 2

I woke up at 2:30 am and got out of bed to go to the bathroom, but my legs wouldn't support me. They felt like mush, so without waking Claire I crawled to the bathroom and managed to get on the toilet, but the magnesium citrate had no effect at all.

My legs felt weird, they were stinging and tingling and they felt cold to touch, and my backside felt like it was sunburned. I had absolutely no idea what was happening to me, but whatever it was, it definitely wasn't right! The scientist in me was dissecting the information every way possible, trying to come up with some alternative that would allow me to teach for the next three days, but my mind could just not comprehend it; it was all so far outside my area of experience. Somehow I managed to crawl back into bed. There was no way I was going back to sleep and no way I was going to disturb Claire. I lay in bed contemplating what on earth could be wrong with me. All the tests that the hospital had performed had ruled things out but I was still no closer to a real diagnosis. I had absolutely no idea what was wrong with me, but I knew that too much stool in my intestine would not cause the inability to walk. I was terrified, in pain, and afraid. I lay awake thinking and praying with all my might for some kind of miracle to occur.

At 5:00 am I felt Claire stirring and woke her and told her that I was still in terrible pain, and that something was seriously wrong with me. It was obvious that I was in no shape to teach any class, so Claire helped to get me dressed and because I was so weak, she called for an ambulance from the fire department to come and take me back to the hospital. She then went in to work to let the staff and students know that the course would have to be rescheduled, and as soon as she was able to get away she came back to the hospital.

In the meantime, at the hospital I was treated again in the emergency room, this time by a different doctor and nurse, and I passed out when a nurse tried to insert an IV line into the back of my hand (I have very protruding veins, and every nurse wants to stick a needle in them, however it isn't as easy as it looks). Finally another nurse got an IV started.

The ER doctor (a new doctor by this time, Dr. Bryce) told me that there was really nothing more that he could do, so he gave me some more of his wonder drug for pain and admitted me to a ward on the third floor where someone would keep me under observation and where I would be seen by more doctors who may or may not run more tests. I was now the property of one Dr. Abraham. After another CT scan (this time without contrast), an abdominal ultrasound and more blood work, there was still no answer to the question of what was wrong with me.

Claire arrived mid morning and while we were talking about how strange this all was, she noticed that my hospital gown was wet! I had urinated and not been aware of it! I had told her that I had passed out when the nurse tried to put the IV in my hand, so we assumed that it had happened while I was passed out, and Claire called in the nurse who got me cleaned up and changed into dry clothing.

Claire and I always travel prepared, for nearly anything, so we took out our Nintendo DS's and played a few games of hearts, rummy, and even some spades, chatting all the while. A couple of hours had passed when Claire noticed that I had wet myself again. This time, while we were trying to figure out what had happened, Claire realized that I wasn't just weak, but I couldn't move my legs at all! We called the nurse, who activated the rapid response team, and the room suddenly filled with people and machines. The prevailing theory expressed out loud was that I might have had a stroke, and when Dr. Abraham arrived and heard that I couldn't move my legs, he called for a neurologist. The neurologist, Dr. Thomas didn't take long to get there. He came in, took one look at me, tested my muscle strength and mobility, and ordered an MRI.

The MRI was extremely difficult for me. I was still under the influence of the good drugs and I kept feeling like I was going to pass out. I was sick to my stomach and the noise was unbearable. Even with all the pain killers, the MRI was still a pain. I could appreciate that it was a phenomenal advance in medicine but it was still a difficult experience.

I think it must have been designed by engineers who came from designing jet engines, air compressors and gas turbines; all pieces of equipment that make very loud noises. This kind of engineer takes the muffler off their vehicle, goes to monster truck rallies and stands next to the power amplifiers at a heavy metal concert. For them, it is all about power and noise. An engine can never be too big, too loud, or too powerful! These people had now turned their attention to medical devices; the only difference being that one doesn't normally want to be inside a jet engine or a gas turbine while it is running. So here I was inside an engineer's dream, a large and powerful heavy metal machine with a three ton magnet in orbit around my head making all kinds of noises that I wasn't sure it was designed to make. It banged, crashed and clanged in accordance with some random pattern, the sole purpose of which seemed to be to worry me, the occupant of the device.

I worried! What if the bearings hadn't been packed with grease? What if it had long passed the most recent planned maintenance date? I could just imagine the three ton magnet coming loose from its housing, smashing through the sheetrock wall and rolling across the cafeteria as people were having breakfast. Meanwhile I had the quiet, reasoned voice of a disembodied person saying things to me, like "another two minutes in this cycle". It seemed that I had entered the twilight zone. It didn't matter what I might have wanted to say, they could talk to me, but I didn't have a microphone to communicate with THEM, and I was nauseous and felt like I was going to pass out, and the only way I could communicate was with a panic button, so I pushed it.

The machine stopped, the magnets ground and shuddered to a halt, I was removed from the machine and a very distraught technician was asking me what was wrong. When I explained that I felt nauseous and like I was going to pass out he told me that I needed to have the MRI done, that it was very important to my diagnosis and treatment. I suggested that if he gave me

15

oxygen to keep me from being light headed, a wet towel for my forehead to help with the nausea, elevated my feet to keep my blood up in my head, and gave me some drug to relax me, I might be able to go through with it. He could see that I was not well so he honored my suggestions. I didn't know if he agreed because I was so persuasive, or because he imagined me throwing up in his machine, but whatever the reason, I got what I asked for and managed to complete the MRI without leaving my stomach's contents all over his equipment. Sometimes you have to stand up for your rights even when you can't actually stand up! I didn't mind standing on principle, but right then I would have been happy to stand on anything.

Dr. Thomas had been observing the MRI, and when he had seen what he needed to see he went back to my hospital room, and arriving there before I did, explained to Claire that I had Transverse Myelitis (TM). For no apparent reason my spine had been attacked by my own immune system causing lesions on my spinal column at the level of thoracic vertebrae T-5 through T-9 and T-11 and T-12.

He explained to her that about 33% of TM patients fully recover, however 33% never recover any capability and the remaining TM patients got some partial recovery. He explained that the treatment was steroids and that to gain more information he would come early in the morning to do a spinal tap.

I arrived back in the room groggy from medication, and Claire took my hand and tried to explain to me what was wrong and what was going to happen but I could barely understand her, and I just kept saying "this is really weird." I guess the drugs had me out of touch with the reality of the situation and I was just not processing the information. Since I was falling asleep, and it was getting quite late, Claire left the hospital promising to

16

be back early in the morning in time for the spinal tap. I don't remember anything else at all about that night.

Day 3

Claire arrived before the neurologist the next morning, thinking that she could be of moral support through the process, which we assumed would be somewhat painful, but luckily (I use that term tongue in cheek) in my case I could not even feel them doing it! Not only was I paralyzed from the chest down, but I also had no feeling at all below the middle of my chest.

At this time I was still experiencing significant chest pain, and in addition I was now experiencing severely debilitating headaches, probably as a result of the spinal tap. We learned later that it might have been possible to avoid these severe headaches if I had remained flat on my back for 6 hours following the spinal tap and ingested some caffeine as well. As it was I suffered headaches for days.

Additionally, I was also still very concerned about the fact that my bowels weren't moving. Since that was the only diagnosis they had come up with in the ER I was still focused on it, so I decided to put myself on a "liquid only" diet to try and avoid adding to the intestinal blockage which I believed was contributing to my pain. As it happened, the stool in my intestines had nothing to do with the pain; the lack of movement in my intestines was due to the lack of signal telling the movement to occur.

We wondered: When Dr. Thomas made his diagnosis of TM, was it communicated to the two ER doctors and the nurses who had cared for me in the ER so that they could diagnose this disorder more quickly should they encounter it in an ER patient in the future?

17

Claire and I spent some time thinking over the events of the previous weeks trying to determine any potential causes of this disorder, and tried to avoid thinking about the future, which looked exceedingly grim. I knew that I would be asked to answer the question "How did you get TM?" and the unstated question would be "How should I avoid it?" My answer would be simple, "I don't have any idea, and nor do my doctors, but because you know me your chances of getting it are practically zero.

There were only two possible reasons I could think for why this might have happened to me. The first was a fall that I had taken when I had done something stupid at home two weeks before.

My wife sometimes thinks that for a seemingly intelligent person, I often act in ways that would belie this fact. We live in a large house on a hill, and at the bottom of our yard there is a fire pit, where we regularly enjoy s'mores with our grandchildren. On one side of the fire pit a gully had been created by rainwater runoff, and Claire, concerned that this gully was a safety hazard, had asked me to fill it partially with dirt and then to line it with concrete to make sure it didn't get any bigger and to keep the grandchildren from falling into it. I had been to the store and bought three bags of cement to do the job. I put the bags of cement in my wheel barrow and proceeded down the hill. Halfway down the hill I did the math, but it was too late. Each bag of cement weighed 80 pounds, the wheelbarrow weighed 30. I, on the other hand weighed about 178. The wheelbarrow was winning the race down the hill, and by the time I had done the math and realized the gravity of the situation, I was losing the battle and gravity was winning. A sensible person would have let go of the wheelbarrow, and let it find its own resting place in our bramble patch, but once again reason escaped me, and so I tried to guide the wheelbarrow towards the fire pit. The wheelbarrow decided that it would prefer to tip over sideways, and as it did, it flipped me over as well. I fell awkwardly on my back and lay there thinking that my wife's thoughts about me were sometimes completely justified.

After a few minutes of telling myself all the things that I could have done to avoid the situation, I realized that I should also have been carrying my cell phone, in case of some emergency, like falling down a hill and then needing to call for help. None of these thoughts, however, were actually helpful in this current situation, so I managed to get to my feet, brush myself off, check that no bones were broken, retrieve the wheelbarrow, mix the cement and finish the job. I took the empty wheelbarrow back up the hill, and got on with my life.

The next morning I expected to be covered in bruises and have stiff and sore muscles, but this didn't happen so I realized that I must be in pretty good shape to bounce back so well after a fall like that. Of course, I didn't tell Claire anything about it, but now, in hindsight, I did wonder if this fall two weeks ago had anything to do with my current situation. One of the possible causes of TM is a spinal shock.

Our second theory had to do with another event, at roughly the same time. A police car had come up our road slowly, not an everyday sight, and stopped just past our neighbor's house. Curious, I walked over and asked the officer what was happening, and he explained that the police had received a 911 call from a man who was lost in the woods behind our house, and the police were trying to find him. I offered to help, and after trudging around in the woods for about an hour, I came back to the house, to find that the police car had left (evidently they had found the missing man) so Claire inspected my bare skin for ticks, which are prevalent in the woods, and found two, which I managed to get off of me before (at least I THINK before) they bit me. One of the possible causes of TM is a tick bite.

Now, TM was my spinal cord disorder, so I decided to do some research. Claire brought my computer in, and the hospital had excellent high speed wireless internet access in every room, so I did a search on "Transverse Myelitis" and found out just how little was known about this uncommon condition. The research indicated that the cause was usually viral, and could be from a hundred different sources (but as much as is possible the doctors had ruled out most of these causes in my case; I hadn't been exposed to a virus or been bitten by a tick (as far as we knew), had a recent vaccination, been exposed to the flu, had aids, herpes or any other one of the usual perpetrators they know can cause TM).

It didn't really matter how it happened or why it happened; these were pointless questions. It happened, and now I was paralyzed from the chest down, and I had to deal with it. I felt like the Black Knight in the movie "Monty Python and the Holy Grail": So what if you cut my legs off, I can still fight and I said to myself, "OK, Keith so what if you are paralyzed, you aren't dead yet!"

The chest pain began to subside somewhat, but I had no control of my bladder so I was catheterized, and I had no intestinal movement; I couldn't concentrate on anything because I still had the terrible headaches.

Claire had brought my MP3 player as well as my computer to the hospital so I started listening to music to distract me from the pain. Suddenly I noticed that my toes were moving to the music. I experimented with my legs, and found that I could slightly move my left leg side to side. It was Day 3, and I felt as though I had been resurrected! I suddenly knew that I was not going to be in the 33% who got no recovery. There was the possibility of recovery, perhaps even of a full recovery, and I sat up and took notice, and did more research on the internet.

Because of the swelling transverse myelitis causes around the spinal cord, it interferes with the nervous system, causing a breakdown in the signals which pass from the brain down the spinal cord to every control system in the body. I had no idea that every human has over 45 miles of nerves in their body and most of them are connected through the spinal cord. Myelenin acts as an insulator between all these electrical wires, and TM strips it away. Without it the wires get crossed, and signals go astray; messages don't get through, and as I had experienced, the effects could be devastating. As the hours went by I discovered that I could now feel pressure and soft touch but I couldn't feel the difference between hot and cold, and when the doctor stuck a pin in me, I could feel no pain!

 Here I was, in the hospital, my senses were gone, and it was getting on my nerves. Something was messing up my central communications superhighway, and it was clearly not as simple as the job I once had testing for telecommunication cable breaks in underground cables.

The company I worked for had installed telephone cables along the side of a highway for emergency phone service (this was WAY before every kid in third grade got a smart phone as a birthday present!). So they designed a cable tester that could pinpoint the exact distance from the testing point to where a cable break had occurred. We would drive along the highway, stop at a phone that didn't work, and send a signal up the cable. The unit would convert the resistance in the cable into a linear distance; we would drive that exact distance, dig a hole, find the cable break, splice it back together, and – presto - normal phone service would be restored! If only it was that easy with my body.

TM is a disorder that affects less than one person in between one and five million, and yes, I was one of these lucky few. Apparently I had a better chance of being struck by lightning twice, or winning the lottery! I also learned that the patients who made the most complete recovery showed significant improvement in the first one to three months, so you can imagine my delight when I saw my toes moving on day 3 and could see movement in my leg as well. This meant that I might be in the first group, the group that gained the fullest and fastest recovery.

Most of my systems appeared to be running fully and properly on automatic: my heart, my lungs, my liver, my kidneys etc. I was grateful beyond belief, yet I was really hoping that one day (soon) I would regain the bowel and bladder control that I had learned over 55 years before. I was now focused on the future, and on seeing what more I could do each day.

With my transfer from the third floor (heavy monitoring) to the eighth floor (less monitoring), we were assigned a case manager, who was responsible for our discharge planning. As near as we could tell at that point, our discharge planning was going to be complex. We were expecting to need home health care, wheelchair rentals, etc., plus the discharge was being planned for someone who lived nearly 3000 miles away, so Claire tried to do what she could to make the case manager's (Kathy's) job easier. She asked some of our friends back home to get the names and phone numbers of organizations that would rent us wheelchairs, provide home health care services, physical therapy, help with bathing, etc., and when she had all that information together, she took it to Kathy, and explained

what she had done. Kathy was grateful but with no discharge
order there was little she could do with it.

Day 4

It took a while for me to feel like drinking anything, much less
eating, but food kept coming, unordered and unwanted. There
was a process to use to get me what I wanted and needed, but
it took us about three days to find out what it was, and in every
hospital we were in, the process differed. In this case, a
dietician would come into the room with an electronic pad, and
offer me choices, most of which I found unappetizing, but on
about day four we were told that there were choices that were
available, but hadn't been offered! Once we knew that, we not
only were able to order what I wanted and needed, but also
order additional snacks to keep my calorie count up while not
adding to my intestinal overload.
I was pleased on the fourth day to look down and see that my
feet, not just my toes, were now moving to the music. Muscle
control was returning slowly from the toes and moving
upwards. I was still on intravenous steroids; something my
research had confirmed was the best thing to do for TM. The
steroids served as an anti-inflammatory drug that would reduce
the lesions around my spinal cord, and also served as an
immune suppressor, which would tell my body to stop
producing the antibodies that were attacking my spinal cord.

My neurologist, Dr. Thomas, continued to visit me every day
and conducted the standard reflex and strength tests and a test
involving a safety pin! He tapped this pin repeatedly on my skin
on various parts of my body, and asked me to tell him whether
it felt sharp or dull. I had absolutely no idea! I couldn't feel
anything at all, so I let him carry on his merry way, until he
reached my upper chest and then suddenly I felt the pain! "Ow,
that hurts!" I realized that it would have been a great time to

get some body piercings, but I can't say that I have ever felt like piercing my body, especially below my rib cage.

The medical staff had inserted a catheter so urine was flowing but so far they hadn't been successful in moving the stool in my intestines. After four days of enemas, laxatives, suppositories and purgatives, I was still seeing nothing from that part of my anatomy. Each day a different doctor or nurse would come in and find some excuse to stick a finger up my backside (oops, sorry! I should have said perform a rectal examination) and at one point I tried to keep track of exactly how many fingers had been in me but lost count when their single digits ran into the double digits! Once again I was glad not to have any feeling in this area.

Any dignity I had ever had, had gone right out the window! It is tough to retain dignity in a hospital gown, and harder still to have any at all in a hospital room. Numerous medical personnel came in at all hours of the day and night to check me out, uncovering my body parts to look at them, poke them, prod at them and prick them, and since I was paralyzed, I was completely dependent on them and Claire for my feeding, changing, medicines and internet service.

Lying in a hospital bed is a great place to reflect on your life, and I had nothing to do now but just that! I had always wanted to be the one in control; I had always been a leader, I loved being in charge, calling the shots, and I always felt I like I should be running everything. As it was, I had been running my own education and consulting company successfully for 27 years. It had been very good to me, and I didn't have to get anyone's permission to take a day off or give myself a bonus just because I wanted or needed one. I must admit that I had a slight attitude problem when I saw idiots in authority, so working for someone else was out of the question, but now my own personal business was everyone else's business; I was completely out of control, and it didn't sit well. In a single day I had regressed about 55 years. I was now a baby with a graying beard. I could just about feed myself, once I could sit up without passing out, but I was baby like in every other way.

As Christians Claire and I had always believed that we were in God's hands, but in our experience, we could usually see where those hands were carrying us! Our lives had just been dealt an enormous blow, and we had no idea what was, or what would be normal from this point on, plus we were nearly 3000 miles away from anyone who seemed to care. Claire's initial reaction was numbness. She set tasks for herself, and one at a time she did them. Her greatest sadness was that she had always had an active prayer life, and for whatever reason, she couldn't get in touch with God. It reminded her of the story of how a man felt so deserted when his life was at its lowest point, and God told the man that it was then that God had been carrying him on his shoulders. We believed that we were in God's hands, but at the moment neither of us could feel it, and she couldn't pray.

Once she got over being numb, she realized that she had to take charge of what life I had under these bizarre circumstances, and that she couldn't just stand by as an observer. From the very beginning she had to keep my spirits up, as well as serve as my arms and legs when I needed something that I couldn't get for myself, which included just about everything, and most importantly, she took responsibility for ensuring that I got the very best medical care ever!

There were some really wonderful staff people in both the ER as well as on the wards, and we relied on them for everything. Neither of us had been hospitalized for well over 35 years, so we were often mystified by everything, the equipment, the procedures, and the staff patterns were all new to us. I know that everyone wanted to do their best, and my experience of the staff in this hospital was they all loved their work, they all wanted to take great care of me, and they were very efficient!

One of the things I had heard of, but had never seen before, was the Computer on Wheels (COW) (but ever since someone on a ward said "Bring that COW into this room" or "Has anyone seen the COW from room 313?" this was no longer acceptable. Computers on Wheels could no longer be referred to as COWs, but had to be something else). In our hospital experience, the computers were called WOWs (workstations on wheels) and we had one in the cubicle in the ER, and one in the room on the ward.

It seemed remarkably efficient. When it was time for medication, the nurse would scan my medical bracelet, and scan the bar code on the medication. This both logged in the computer that I had taken the medication, as well as that I was the correct patient, and that the medication being given was in fact the correct medication and in the correct dose as that which had been ordered for me. When they took my vital signs, they were entered directly into the data base, and whenever a doctor needed to review my records, test results, or treatment history, it was all instantaneously available. I didn't realize until later what this meant in terms of the amount of hands on patient care I would receive. The nursing staff was often in our room, and each person was warm, friendly, and genuinely caring.

Early on we started a diary which we called our "Illness Diary" where we documented the events of every day, and at about day 25 we realized that we had been through a lot, and had learned a few things about the health care system, about being a patient, and about being an advocate for someone ill, and we felt that they were important enough to add to this book as lessons for those in the health care system, for patients, for family and for friends.

We share them at the end of the book in the hopes that they will be the starting point for a dialogue that will dramatically improve the quality of our health care. We hope that they will also serve as a guide for patients who are capable of participating in their own recovery, because the final and most important lesson is that everyone must be prepared to take responsibility for their own recovery. These lessons are also a guide for the friends and family of patients to help them serve as advocates for their loved ones.

Chapter 2 – In the Hospital

Looking at it, life in a hospital bed might seem cool! No responsibilities, you get to sleep all day, people bring you your food and if you're lucky, you might actually get to choose your meals from a menu, almost like in a restaurant! People come to visit you and bring you flowers, or better yet more food, and you can read all day, or watch television, and no one will think you're lazy. But it is never as good as you think it's going to be, and isn't nearly as much fun as living life outside the hospital.

If you have ever visited someone in the hospital you know that people's health becomes the primary focus of every conversation. I suddenly realized that I had always treated my health as a hygiene factor, something I took for granted when I had it, but now that I didn't have it, it dominated my whole life. When I went to the ER on Day 1, Claire told our children that we thought that I had food poisoning. On Day 2 we had to tell our children, Claire's parents, my mother, as well as our siblings and a few very close friends that it was a bit more serious than that. On Day 3 we posted the information on Facebook, notifying the immediate world, friends, co-workers, basically everyone we knew that I was down for the count, with no assurance that I would ever rise again.

Now my whole world was contained within the four walls of a hospital room. I had one very valuable window to the outside, to family and friends: a laptop computer connected to the world outside. Now my real world had become virtual, and the virtual world had become real. Thanks to internet access, my friends and family appeared on my screen, broadcasting from the other side of the country, and even the other side of the world, thanks to Skype, and floods of encouraging words poured in through posts to our favorite social network. In the meantime, there I was another strange case for Doctor House.

I remember waking up one morning overcome with sadness because I couldn't hug my grandchildren. We were separated by three time zones, a few great lakes, and a whole bunch of states, and I felt overwhelmed, so I asked everyone who loved me to send me photographs that I could post in my room so that I could see their faces every day, and I was amazed at the response that I got. Photos arrived from our biological family, our church family and our friends, and some people wrote "get well" messages on the back of their photos. It was wonderful to know that people were thinking of us!

It was tough to be so far from family and friends. Everyone was very concerned and wanted to know what they could do to help; several people offered to fly out to San Francisco and help us, but the reality was that there was not much for them to do. The doctors and nurses were doing everything they could for me, and Claire was there to be my advocate and deal with the inevitable challenges that are part of health care in America today. Facebook became our preferred method of connecting with everyone since with one message, which Claire could copy from her page and then paste on mine, we communicated with hundreds of people, sometimes multiple times a day, and they could post their own comments of encouragement, always encouragement. It made us feel not quite so alone when we were so far away! We were connected, and it made our experience a bit less lonely.

The third day after I had been admitted to the hospital it became very clear that we were not flying home on the date we had originally planned. Reality was beginning to sink in. We didn't know what our future would look like, or even when the rest of our life would begin. Claire called the airline and cancelled our return flight.

I am a planner; I love to plan, I teach planning, I admire people with plans, I respect schedules, and I get paid for measuring performance to plan. Now my life was out of control; I didn't have a plan and this was getting on the last few nerves I had that were still communicating with my brain. I had to have a plan; there had to be a way forward. I had to get well; I had to get back to my family and friends. I had to get back to work. I couldn't just lie here and let my life be defined by a functional abnormality or some medical disorder.

I had Transverse Myelitis, my spinal column was the battlefield between my body's natural defense forces and a perceived invader, and I wasn't able to do anything except lie there and imagine the kinds of havoc that the collateral damage and friendly fire would have. I did try a cease fire order; my brain specifically instructed the opposing forces to lay down their weapons and leave the battlefield, but it was already too late. Communications were down, the wires were crossed, and both sides were too busy fighting to stop and listen anyway.

Day 4 (Continued)

It was Friday morning, and a nurse rolled in a scale, and said "Jump up on the scale, I need to weigh you." I looked at Claire, she looked at me, and we both turned to the nurse. Claire said "He's paralyzed! He can't move!" This happened several times. A nurse (always a new nurse) would ask "Have you been up and gone to the bathroom yet?" or "Did you get up and brush your teeth?" "Did you take your shower?" It sure was nice when the shift turnover happened in our room, and we knew that at least for that shift, we wouldn't have to say out loud that fearsome word "paralyzed".

A nurse friend of ours told us that often at shift start she had to hit the ground running, and barely had time to find out which patients were hers before some crisis occurred and she had to get to work, so we are sensitive to the fact that not every nurse on every shift had the time to read up on my condition, but Sally Franz, who wrote the book "Scrambled Leggs" after her own ordeal with TM had a similar experience, and found herself railing "read the chart"

It was time to make some new plans. OK, so we were not flying home on schedule, but that didn't mean that we couldn't have a plan! I was going to get out of bed, get in a wheelchair, get started on physical therapy and start repairing the carnage that had been wreaked in my spinal column, so I was thrilled when a physical therapist came in to work with me.

Her first plan was to help me transfer to a wheelchair. I felt confident that I could do it, after all I could still use my arms, and my upper body was still strong so how difficult could it be? I had seen wheelchair athletes in Special Olympics doing amazing things in their wheelchairs, so obviously it would be easy for me, with my good upper body strength, to simply slide across a board, and move from my bed to the wheelchair.

I sat up in bed, and as I tried to slide across the board into the wheelchair, I passed out.

This was definitely not in my plan! I had assumed that it would be simple but it was say more than that. Something was screwed up. As it happens, it was one of those many autonomic functions that we take for granted. I didn't know what happened in a person's body to regulate and adjust blood pressure, much less that it could be compromised, but this mechanism was essential for me to safely sit up or stand up, much less function in vertical mode, and it was broken. A team of people streamed in, got me back into bed, and called for the doctor who ordered another MRI, this time of my head, and I began to realize just how much work would be required just to get me into a position where I could even start physical therapy. I suddenly realized that this might be "it"! That my life, from now on, might be so totally and radically different from what it had been that it might be unrecognizable. There were no indications that I would ever be able to sit up in a chair, much less ever walk again, and now I was totally depressed and Claire was devastated.

From my previous MRI experience, I knew what was required, so I told the nurse who was getting me ready "I need Ativan (the drug used to relax me), oxygen, and an icepack on my head." Everyone bustled around and got it all for me right away, and I was off!

As they wheeled me away for the MRI of my head, Dr. Abraham came into the room, and Claire was obviously distressed. He asked her how she was, and she told him that she could handle anything, that if I never walked again she could accept that, but that what she couldn't handle was seeing me so depressed. Later that afternoon a social worker stopped by our room to talk with us. She told us that Dr. Abraham had asked her to stop by and speak with us, in particular with Claire, because he could see that she was in distress. That act meant everything to us! As it happened, by the time she arrived we were back on an even keel, and were feeling much more positive, but the fact that the Doctor not only noticed, but also called someone to come see us, was really thoughtful!

At 11:00 we were visited by a doctor who specialized in rehabilitation therapy. Dr. Romano told us that there was an acute (I really thought he said "there was a cute") rehabilitation facility in the city that specialized in spinal cord injuries and disorders, and he strongly suggested that we try and get transferred to this unit. He told us that I was an "excellent" candidate for rehab because of my attitude and my strength, and that I would have to be prepared to do three hours of physical therapy every day. I was very motivated to do this, but Claire, ever the pragmatist, explained to him that it all depended on insurance company (our particular insurance company was GIC) approval. He assured us that he would help defend the recommendation!

Claire had to figure out who to call to let them know that I was in the hospital, out of our home region, perhaps in it for the long haul, and "oh, by the way," wanted to go to a rehab unit that might not be on their "approved list", so she started the ball rolling and got the phone number of the California regional office of GIC. When she called them, they didn't even have a record of my admission, despite it being day 4 of our ordeal, and my third day as an admitted patient. She found out what GIC required as proof of admission, and then went to the hospital admissions office and explained what was needed. The financial management person in the hospital admissions office showed her a copy of the fax that had already been sent to GIC that day, with all the required information, and explained that "sometimes it takes a while for the information to get 'into the system'".

That afternoon Belinda Knowles, a representative from the rehab center Dr. Romano had recommended, came to visit with us to explain about the treatment available and to show us brochures about the acute rehab unit. Between Dr. Romano, Belinda, and the pictures of this newly renovated acute rehabilitation unit, we were sold on the place! We were ready! Small problem: the rehab unit was right in the heart of San Francisco, this was the middle of summer and the peak period for gouging tourists, and even the cheap hotel rooms were ridiculously priced, far too expensive for Claire to stay nearby. Claire went on line to try to figure out where she might be able to stay, but could find only a couple of hotels that were reasonable, and we were very worried.

It isn't often the case, I imagine, but occasionally I would guess hospitals got patients visiting from somewhere else, in our case, nearly 3000 miles away, and in those instances, there might also be a family member, or more than one family member, frightened, in an unfamiliar area, with no plan for how to function in this very new, strange environment. In our case, Claire was an extremely resourceful person, but she also knew that there was plenty she didn't know about the area. The first thing she encountered, was that the websites offering information about hotels all assumed you knew exactly where you were going! For example, San Francisco hotels are divided into geographic areas such as Union Square, Fisherman's Wharf, Civic Center, East Bay, etc. Well, none of that meant anything to us, so she had to ask the nurses which of those areas the rehab unit was in. They didn't know! No one had a map of course, and a map wouldn't necessarily have had the same designated areas as the website Claire was looking at, so one nurse called her husband, and he directed her to a website that had hotels by hospitals, which was extremely helpful! It also brought to the nurses' attention that we were worried about a place for Claire to stay, and so she offered Claire a cot in my room beginning immediately! What a blessing!

Now we are not poor, by any means, but we also hadn't budgeted for a lengthy hotel stay that was now not going to be a business expense, much less reimbursable by the client, and being self employed, I was not only not getting paid, but possibly would never work again, so you can imagine how much of a blessing it really was! That "above and beyond" behavior characterized most of the staff at this particular hospital. We were to find that this wasn't universally true.

When we mentioned our concern about a hotel in close proximity to the rehab center, Belinda told Claire that she would be able to stay on a cot in my room until she found something else, which was a huge relief, so now everything was decided on our part, and it was just a question of waiting to see if we could get the approval to transfer from the hospital to rehab from GIC.

At this point we discovered a major flaw in the healthcare system in America today. People get sick at all times of the day or night, but insurance companies keep office hours. Hospitals try to get patients out of the facilities for the weekends, and on Friday afternoon it was decided by the entire medical team that I would be better off in rehab, I was ready for rehab, and rehab wanted me. Given that, the best and most cost effective decision would have been to transfer me immediately. Unfortunately, the system doesn't move at that speed. Transfers don't happen quickly, certainly not quickly enough for me! My fast track recovery was stuck in the slow lane as the weekend passed me by. Claire made sure that we got what we wanted by leaving no stone unturned to get it, but we were helpless when there was no one at the other end of the phone, and we spent a lot of time in a holding pattern.

If you want a patient to get better, you have to keep him/her motivated and moving in a positive direction. To do that, the road must be clear of obstacles preventing their recovery at all times, and that means that people must be available to make decisions and execute plans at any time, and they must be very efficient and very effective at doing it.

My wife is a very smart and capable woman. She retired from the Navy in 1998, and she discovered many ways to get people to do things that they really didn't want to do. She knows innately how to deal with bureaucrats, she can spot red tape a mile off, and she can pinpoint the exact place that a business process is flawed, and how it could be corrected. She can sense when she is being given the run around, and she knows how to cut through it and get results. Among many other things this is one of her qualities that I most admire, and rely on, even though from time to time I see the impact in the fallen bodies behind her. I have yet to develop the skill, patience, and diplomacy to deal with bureaucracy. She does it with ease. Unfortunately, during this period of our lives she would have to do it a lot!

Fortunately my time was not completely wasted. I had been selected to present a paper with a co-worker from a client company at an upcoming conference, and the deadline for submitting the final presentation was upon us, so we needed to get together and review it. Debbie agreed to come to my hospital room so that we could work on the presentation together. She was the first person I had seen besides Claire who was not a part of the health care system. She was in civilian clothes, cheerful and smiling, full of energy and enthusiasm, and it was a great meeting, if under rather bizarre circumstances, and we were able to work, uninterrupted, until we were satisfied with the end result.

During Debbie's visit, a volunteer came by and asked if she could talk with us for a few minutes about our stay! Claire stepped out of the room with her, and had a wonderful opportunity to share with someone our feelings about the terrific care we had received! Our experiences and the names of the nurses and doctors were fresh in our minds, and so she was readily able to mention each one by name, and what specifically that person had done to make our stay more positive! The volunteer wrote rapidly as Claire gave her name after name of someone who had made a dramatic and significant difference in the quality of our lives, and specifically what that person had done. It was wonderful to be able to share that information with someone so that it could hopefully be used to reward those people for their hard and well appreciated efforts!

By the end of the day I noticed that I had some additional movement in my left leg. I could raise it a little off the bed and could also move it from side to side, and the oppressive pain across my rib cage and my intense headache had also decreased, so that made things more cheerful and at the end of the day I felt far more optimistic than ever before.

I had a great private room in the hospital, and my bed was close to the window. I had a great view of the hills surrounding the peninsula, and in the evening as the sun went down there was a good view of three bright planets over the hills. I looked this up on the internet and discovered that this was a rare alignment of Jupiter, Saturn and Uranus. (I also discovered that if we had been able to see it, Pluto was also in this alignment, but Pluto, having recently been downgraded from a planet to a dwarf planet, didn't count anymore.) I was hoping that this was a sign from heaven, that my situation was temporary, and that I needed to keep my planets in order. I renamed the three planets: God, the Power of Prayer, and Positive Attitude, and I was convinced that this trinity would be the key to my recovery.

Day 5

Claire woke up at 3:00 am in an absolute panic! She suddenly realized that we had a car parked in Boston at the airport! We had pre-paid for our five days of parking but if we left the car there until we could go get it, we would truly be broke! So when she came in to the hospital in the morning we called our daughter and let her know that there was something truly significant that she could do to help! After giving her all the details and getting her promise that she and her husband would take care of it, we relaxed. One crisis averted! It was the first of many.

Then Claire told me of the success she had had the evening before, buying all the things that we needed to have in rehab. Belinda had given us a list of things that I needed, including a bunch of clothes I didn't have with me! Remember, our original plan was to fly in, teach for three days and then fly home, but now we had watched as that plan took off without us, and here we were, unsure how long it would be before we could catch a new plan out of here. All that we DID know was that we wanted to go to rehab for as long as it took to get me back on my feet or into a wheelchair and capable of some kind of independent living. This might be a week, a month, a few months or a year; we had no idea. We had each brought enough clothes for 3 days of work, as well as workout clothes and a few casual clothes, not enough for a month in a rehab unit. So Claire was as resourceful as ever, and had taken care of things, as she does so well; I was nearly outfitted for rehab.

My second attempt at physical therapy was more successful, and during this session I managed to sit up straight on the side of the bed without passing out, and scoot to the left and right on the bed, and even managed to use my legs to support some of my weight. I was high as a kite! This was a piece of cake! I was going to be walking soon!

In the afternoon we had a visit from a friend, Sharon, who had actually driven for over three hours to be with us. It was so great to see her! She and her husband had been with us on a business trip to China in 2000 and we had been friends ever since. He had even followed in my footsteps, rising to the elevated position of 2010 President of the volunteer society of which I had been President in 1991. In some respects I blamed myself for his folly. Being the President of a volunteer organization is a lot of work, and the pay is lousy (nothing), but I had encouraged him to become a speaker at one of their international conferences, and the rest is history! He rose through the ranks as a bright shining star. Unfortunately, he was away at yet another weekend meeting, so Sharon had decided to make the trip and spend some time with us. She brought me a teddy bear which became my constant companion, and I named the bear Karla. Karla had a prominent position in each of my rooms, along with all the photographs I had received.

This adds yet another small irk that we had to contend with, that of the revolving beds. When I was admitted to the hospital on day two of my ordeal I was sent to the third floor, and was in a room there where I was hooked up to all kinds of monitoring devices. When they realized that I didn't really need to be monitored so closely, I was sent to the eighth floor, and then a day later, I was sent to the seventh floor.

With the move to the seventh floor we were assigned another case manager, Candy, who stuck with us every second and fought hard for us. Claire explained to her that she had given all the information to Kathy, and Candy said that she would get it from her, and follow up. She did, all the way through the remainder of our stay.

Claire's had checked out of our original hotel since it was costing her $30 in taxi fare each way to and from the hospital, and checked into a less expensive hotel within walking distance of the hospital. She had left two suitcases with the staff at the original hotel, and so while Sharon was there with her car, she and Sharon left to go and retrieve the suitcases and to buy the final few things that I needed for rehab.

When they returned from their excursion I could see that Claire looked sad and I couldn't understand why, until she admitted that she had lost my wedding ring, which I had given her for safe keeping when I went for the MRI. She had been wearing my ring on her finger but it had fallen off somewhere in her travels, and she was upset, and very sad. I told her that it didn't matter, as long as we were still together a ring could always be replaced, and sure enough, Claire went online that very evening, and we picked out some matching rings nearly identical to the one she had lost. We ordered them to be delivered to our home, and although we still didn't know when exactly we would get to be there to open the box and put them on, we were happy.

Day 6

Sunday was a mixed day. The nurses gave me a bed bath and washed my hair with this terrific baggie thing that they nuke and then put on your head, and massage around! No rinsing is required, and for the first time in six days, I felt refreshed! Claire followed all of this by giving me a massage. My left leg showed some more movement, but my right leg was still totally unresponsive; my brain was sending signals telling it to move and it responded like a teenager in the morning, with a mind of its own, and not afraid to disobey orders.

I was also still concerned that I hadn't had a bowel movement for six days, and I knew this could neither be normal nor healthy. If my intestine was full of stool on Tuesday (and since then I had been downing prune juice, warm prune juice, warm prune juice mixed with pineapple juice, laxatives, stool softeners, and magnesium citrate, and had tried enemas, suppositories, and had people sticking fingers in my backside) what in the world was going on in there on day 6! I thought that my bowel must have been talking to my right leg, and that they both had adopted a program of non co-operation. I know that my bladder would have been over full except that it had a tube stuck in it through my private parts, and so I was wondering if I should call the guy who emptied our septic system and have him bring his truck and use his suction hose to help things along. No one else seemed to be concerned however, so we just kept rolling along!

As alone as we were, so far from friends and family, we knew that there were people who cared, and that made everything more bearable, but we were so dependent on others it was very difficult for us; we had always been people on whom others could rely! We were awash in a sea of darkness, the future was so uncertain, and we were dependent on the mercy of strangers who had no more requirement to care for us than that defined by their simple duty, and yet they chose to take on our fight, to care for us, and to go above and beyond the call of duty! We were unbelievably grateful that they chose to value us and care about what happened with and to us, and to act accordingly!

It was now time for a serious discussion about what our short and medium term plans would be. We now knew that the road ahead would be long and difficult. We knew that there was the distinct possibility that I might not work for another 6 months if ever, although I was confident that I could still teach, even if it was in a wheelchair.

We made some important decisions including the decision to postpone any decision about the August class I was scheduled to teach until I had been in rehab for 10 days; we agreed to contact another good friend in case I needed to have her take over my classes, and we made some serious decisions about finances.

My wife is retired and she gets her monthly Navy pension and her Social Security payment each month. I am self employed and my income is used to pay 100% of my expenses, 50% of our joint expenses and 75% of our house expenses (Claire and I have a somewhat complicated financial arrangement, she has her money, I have my money and we have our money. This works out fine for me. She does all the bookkeeping and keeps things straight; taking care of all the bills, freeing me up to do more of the household maintenance chores).

My business income has enabled us to do some things we would not normally have been able to do. In 2005, after a long discussion we moved into a much larger house than we needed with the agreement that I would pay for 75% of the monthly expenses related directly to the house. We had way more space than we could justify for two people, but we didn't see utilization as the important measure; we saw that we needed the capacity to have our family around us.

We were thrilled when our first grandchild was born, have been equally happy when the other four were delivered, and are excited to know that the sixth is on order and coming next year. Our family keeps getting bigger, and our house is the only place we can all get together and sit down at the ever expanding table, so even though we didn't need it, we bought a really big house, and then we built an extension!

We sold our condo in Fort Lauderdale at the right time, before the market crashed, so we had a chunk of money that we invested in the construction of an indoor pool which we attached to our house. We live in New Hampshire and the idea of swimming year round seemed very decadent but once again it wasn't just for us; we thought the grandchildren might enjoy it. As it happens, it is the one thing that they always agree on. Given a choice of things to do they always select swimming, and they never want to get out of the pool. Apart from the oldest two who already knew how to swim, the other grandchildren have all learned how to swim in our pool, even the 4 year old, and they are very good swimmers. The downside is the heating bill. They prefer the pool to be warm (they will live with 80 degrees, but far prefer 84 degrees) and so we require 2000 gallons of propane every year to heat our house and the pool. With all of this, we have three large monthly budget line items: mortgage, taxes and propane. These are all house expenses and consequently 75% mine, since it was my decision to go the "big house" route.

This would all now be in serious jeopardy if I was disabled, so it was time to let the family know what the future looked like. We developed a budget based on absolute minimum requirements, and we were clearly looking at a very different lifestyle. Using my wife's fixed pension income we could stay in the house, as long as we:
Didn't go out to eat or shop for anything more than groceries, closed the pool and the hot tub, and didn't do anything fun other than play board games and watch one of the 1000 or so DVDs we owned. It was time to tell the family the good times might be coming to an end. We composed an email and sent it to them saying basically that if dad was disabled and unable to work, life would look pretty different for us and for them.

All this thinking had made my brain hurt, and not only did I have a headache, but also the pain in my rib cage was still a 6. I refused to take the narcotics they had readily available, and instead, asked for an alternative route to pain management. I asked for Lidocaine patches for my rib pain and Tylenol for my headache. This had some limited effect, but it was usually manageable and at least I wasn't throwing up every 15 minutes, but as the day wore on, the pain got worse, and I wasn't able to do anything when the physical therapist came for my session.

My blood pressure dropped like a stone when I sat up, and I was very weak.

I was certainly not at my best, when I had another visitor; a student of mine, who had graduated through my teaching program, achieved his certification, and had kept in touch afterwards. He had called and told us that he would bring us some homemade truffles! Being a genuine chocoholic, I was eager for his visit, and it was uplifting just when I needed uplifting, when he came by with a box of his nearly world famous Vidamor Chocolate truffles!

Claire took him out for a cup of coffee as I was not quite energetic enough for socializing, and finally as I lay there feeling sorry for myself, the intestinal dam broke and suddenly there was sh*t everywhere, literally! Like I said, a mixed day!

Day 7

It was Monday, the day we hoped to hear a decision about rehab. I woke up strong and raring to go, and I detected some movement from my right leg; it wasn't ready to get up and get going, but at least it showed some signs that it might still be alive! I still had considerable pain, so using Lidocaine patches on my ribs and Tylenol and Salonpas patches (an over the counter pain patch) on my forehead I managed to make the pain bearable (I looked pretty silly, but I could function).

The Foley catheter was removed and replaced with a condom catheter in preparation for my hoped for transfer, and all morning we waited for some word to come from GIC.

Late in the morning we were visited by our hospital case manager, Candy, who told us that GIC wanted an additional 26 pages of documentation. This was making her mad as hell, but she assured us that she was on the case! She was a tiny woman, but she made it clear to us that she was not one to argue with and that there was no way that she was going to lose this fight. She was in our corner and she would win this for us. She was an inspiration and we felt confident that she could do what she said. She was as good as her word. She had argued our case and won, so by 2:15 pm the discharge papers were signed, the ambulance arrived and we were ready to go to the rehab center.

This presented us with another small problem. Claire and I come to California to teach every month, and we always stay at the same hotel, so we have a great arrangement with them. We are able to leave two suitcases with them between our trips, so we don't always have to haul four suitcases around with us. Now, four suitcases might sound a bit excessive, but one half of one suitcase is taken up by a special pillow that Claire has to alleviate the symptoms of Gastroesophageal Reflux Disease (GERD) and Gastritis. One quarter of a suitcase is taken up by my Continuous Positive Airway Pressure (CPAP) machine (yes, as if TM is not enough when added to atonic seizures, I also have sleep apnea), and the last quarter of one suitcase is taken up with teaching materials for the class that we are scheduled to teach. One suitcase is used for my business clothes and shoes, one for Claire's clothes and shoes, and one for our workout gear, which includes an underwater walkman, a swimming tether, bathing suits, and gym shoes, toiletries, etc. So yes, we travel heavy.

Now we had added this long list of things that I needed for rehab, so Claire had all four suitcases, as well as two carry-on bags each with computers etc. in my hospital room. Once she had gotten out the things I would need for rehab, we no longer needed access to the suitcases, but there was no place to put them, so we had stashed them behind the bed. It wasn't a problem here in this hospital, but it became a big problem later, especially when Claire had to manage moving them on her own.

Chapter 3 - In Rehab

Day 7 (Continued)

The rehab center was a totally different world from a regular hospital ward, although it was a part of a hospital so a lot of the same things applied. It was obvious from the moment we arrived that these people were serious about "fixing" you. During the previous year they had put the whole unit through some serious rehab of its own, to the tune of $92 million. My room looked like a room in a health spa or a hotel, but for disabled people, and it had an inverted train track in the ceiling going all round the room and into the bathroom. In the corner of the room was a mechanical crane with attachments turning it into some kind of robotic device which could be used to move people around supported by the overhead tracks. I wondered if they would be using this to move me around, rather like a side of beef in an abattoir. In my work I had seen many examples of systems like this for moving "stuff" around factories, but hadn't considered using it to haul people as well!

A very pleasant young man came into my room to help me get settled. He introduced himself as Aaron, and handed me a large notebook, and handed Claire a form asking her to document all the personal items that we had in our possession. This was a daunting task. At this point we were still in possession of all the things that we needed for our work in California, plus all the additional things that Claire had purchased for my use since arriving, so our list was far longer than the one page pre-printed form that he gave us. We had all our electronic toys: we each had our own laptop, MP3 player (three in total, since I had two); portable game players, cell phones, phone chargers, two cameras, two external hard drives and Claire had her Kindle. We also had an assortment of memory sticks and power supplies. We don't travel light, and everything we had was with us.

While I am very clear that not everyone arrives at rehab with four suitcases, four carry-on bags, and a host of electronics, a pre-printed form will not always fit every need, so if it's going to be used, there really should be a way to amend it so it could be used effectively. In our case, it was completely unworkable, and that should have been obvious from the beginning when the admissions nurse saw us arrive with all our "stuff". What we really needed was a whole legal pad! Claire was going to be in my room until she found a hotel and we had nowhere else to put stuff, so she made a valiant attempt to record everything on the form.

Policies are necessary, I get that, but it is my theory that behind every rule and every policy ever written lies an event that occurred once that caused a problem, thereby requiring a rule or a policy to ensure it never happened again. The problem with this, is that there are so many policies, that no one can get their arms around all of them, and some become pro-forma, that is without any real value.

The "itemize your belongings" form was a perfect example. Once Claire had done her best to document all of our possessions on this one page pre-printed form, there was a column where someone from the rehab unit was supposed to verify that we did indeed have all the things that we said we had, and then we were both to sign it, and presumably one copy would remain with me, and the second with the hospital staff. In all the days we were at the rehab unit, that second step never occurred, in fact, when Claire packed to leave rehab, she still had the completed form, intact, in her possession.

We were a little nervous about all our electronics, and in each room there was one closet with a combination lock on it. Unfortunately, no one volunteered to tell us how to program it. I guess there wasn't a checklist for the staff so that they could verify that they had made us aware of all the things we could take advantage of. When Claire did finally ask about using the closet lock, she did get the staff to find the keys to program it.

Our room was tastefully decorated with sea foam green walls and we had a great view of the downtown area from our windows. It felt more like being in a hotel than a hospital. We even had a flat screen high definition television! Aaron set me up with dinner, ordered of course without consideration of my tastes, and he answered a lot of our questions and left us alone for the evening, which was actually a welcome change. Fortunately, the hospital cafeteria was still open, and so Claire was able to get something to eat.

After supper Claire unpacked, put everything we would need away, and then repacked everything we wouldn't be using for a while into two of the suitcases, then put those full suitcases inside the two empty suitcases, thereby reducing our footprint by nearly one-half. Of course, this made everything more difficult when I would decide that there was something she had packed away that I actually needed! She found a space to stash the suitcases and carry-on bags, and then she got to relax. While she was doing this, I was productively occupied. She had set up my computer for me and I began to try to communicate with our friends and family to give them our new address and the phone number of our rehab suite! What did I discover???? We didn't have internet access! In this brand new rehab center, they had not installed wireless internet access. They had installed four Ethernet ports in each room, but of course in this day and age we didn't travel with Ethernet cables (that would of course lead to either starting suitcase #5 or taking bigger heavier suitcases). The hospital staff didn't have Ethernet cables for us to use either. The internet was our lifeline to our friends, family and the whole world outside of this room, and our lifeline was dead. Additionally, as a self employed person, I had to stay in touch with clients. We were posting Facebook updates on a daily basis, sometimes more often than that, plus we had to pay our bills, I had to carry on my business, we had to read and respond to emails from clients and we needed to research TM! It wasn't like we wanted to cruise porn sites or play Farm Town all day!

I know that not all patients, in fact, probably a minimum number of patients, will arrive as well equipped as we were for communicating with the outside world, but one of the highlights of our days in the first hospital were the times we got to Skype with our family and friends. We didn't realize how fortunate we were to have high speed wireless access in the initial hospital all the time. We were struck dumb by our inability to connect here in rehab. We were told with a smile that there was a computer in the activity room for patients to use. Excuse me, I was paralyzed and immobile, so that wasn't going to help!

Item #1 on the following day's "To Do" list: Buy Ethernet cables!

As promised, the staff delivered a fold up cot for Claire to sleep on, so she rearranged the furniture to allow room for it, set it up next to the windows, changed into workout pants and a t-shirt, we said our prayers, and she climbed into her little bed.

It didn't turn out to be exactly the night she had hoped for. Even though we were in rehab and not in the "hospital", there was still a lot of "stuff" that happened at night, all of which required light and made noise. Claire is an extremely light sleeper; she says it is because she is a "mother" and always has to listen for her children, and in the day time she can hear a gnat fart at 50 meters, so every single sound, and there were many, woke her up. She was also always worried that I would need something, and sometimes I did, so she was, among other things, my night nurse. Every four hours someone came in to take my vital signs, every shift change I had to be "seen", at 5:00 am the vampires arrived to suck my blood, then there were meds, and often the nurse forgot to close the door, so there was a lot of light and noise, but we were together, and that was lovely!

Day 8

My wife became very focused on her mission as my advocate: correct the problem of not having internet. Not having access was unacceptable, so Claire disappeared to deal with the issue. She asked a member of the staff where there was an office supply store within walking distance. There wasn't one. OK....how about a drug store? That there was, about nine blocks away, nine San Francisco Blocks! Have you ever tried to walk around San Francisco? Claire is, among other things, disabled from a fall she had while in the military, and has really bad knees, so it didn't take long for San Francisco to do her in, but she valiantly set off, and sure enough, found us Ethernet cables! She was so pleased!

My new occupational therapist came in and introduced herself. Her name was Miriam, and she would be with me as my primary occupational therapist for my entire rehabilitation. She helped me to sit up and get dressed, and checked out my movement. I had good movement in my left leg, but my right leg was still on strike, so simple things like putting on socks were neither quick nor easy. She insisted that I wear socks with non-slip soles whenever I was up, and since "up" was what I really wanted, non-slip socks it was! She even gave me a tool to help me hold my leg in position while I put my socks on. I had no idea that such a device existed, and I later found out how useful it could be for other purposes then that for which it was intended. It consisted of two strong fabric loops connected by a rigid connector about two and a half feet long. I thought she was pulling my leg, and it turned out that that was exactly what she wanted me to do with it. One circle went around my foot, and the other circle was in my hand. I could then use my hand to pull my foot up to put on my sock! It was quite clever. Later I tried to search for it on the Internet, but none of the results showed anything like the object she just gave to me. She also gave me something called a "helping hand", a 26 inch long grabber that you could use for all kinds of purposes, but was designed to help you reach things that were out of your normal reach or were down on the floor. Thus began my occupational therapy.

Following my 45 minutes with Miriam, my new physical therapist came in and introduced herself. Her name was Karen, and I shared with her that I was watching my muscles disappear on a daily basis and I needed to get back to exercises that would kick start building back my muscle strength. I was still in some pain, my blood pressure still dropped like a stone whenever I sat up, and both Miriam and Karen agreed that I was in no fit shape to do much of anything yet. It was really depressing and I started really worrying that I might never recover.

Claire came back from her mission with Ethernet cables, one for each of us, and we set about getting connected! Ethernet ports to the left of us, Ethernet ports to the right of us, Ethernet ports everywhere, and not a one would work! Were we doing something wrong? We didn't think so, so Claire set out to instill a sense of urgency in the powers that be to get us online, and returned from her mission with a vague promise from someone that "he would look into it". When she came back and saw that

I was feeling discouraged, she handed me a pad of paper and a pencil, and said "Write down all the things that you can do today that you couldn't do on July 21st" (day 2). It had been exactly one week since the pain had hit me and six days since I had been completely paralyzed without sensation in my body from my chest down. In the space of one week I could now: move the toes on both legs; circle the ankles on both legs; raise my left leg to my chest; roll over onto either side; dress myself; wash my body; move my knees together and apart; sit up in bed without passing out; scoot a few inches to the right and left when sitting up; eat real food and defecate (with a little help). Making this list, I realized how far I had come, and I began to look at things in a far more positive way. Now I made a list of the things that I could do on July 21st that I couldn't do now, but there was only one thing on that list, connect to the internet!

My next visit was from Dr. Matthews, who performed a series of muscle tests, examined me and asked if I had any pain. I told him that I did, and so he ordered some pain medication. He asked if I had any nausea, and when I said yes he ordered some anti-nausea medication. I suddenly understood the magic that is modern medicine: To some doctors, the solution to any medical problem is found in a bottle of pharmaceuticals. I waited breathlessly for the bottle that had the cure for TM, but then I realized that there were so few patients with it that it wasn't a big enough market for any company to fund and do the research necessary to bring a drug to cure it to market.

Later in the day I had a visit from a speech therapist. This was a mandatory part of the evaluation for any new patient, and so she asked me what day it was, to which I replied that it was Tuesday, July 27th and that while the time was actually 1:00 pm Pacific Standard Time, the time on the television display appeared to be off by about 11 hours. I also told her that given that it was the 21st century, one would think that a rehab center that had just spent $92million on renovations could and should have installed wireless routers throughout the building. She put a check mark on her clip board: "No cognitive impairment" and asked me if I would like some help with my speech. I said "Sure! I am giving one in October, would you like to write it for me?" She explained that she meant my "diction", and I said "You mean like so like I can talk like a valley girl, huh?" She put another check on her clipboard: "No speech therapy required".

After she left, I had a visit from the neuropsychologist, Dr. Bradley. He was a very pleasant man who was concerned about my mental state. I told him that I was going nuts because I couldn't access the Internet, and he seemed very sympathetic to my problem (of course, he is a neuropsychologist, so that is a part of the job description). He told me that he would do what he could to rectify the situation, but reminded me that while it might be very important for me to be able to connect, my main focus had to be on getting well. I promised if I could connect, then I would be happy to switch off, but at the moment I felt that I needed my electronic lifeline to maintain my sanity. After this flood of visitors completed their evaluations we were left alone for the evening, and since we still had no internet access, we watched our only DVD on my computer.

Before going to bed on her little cot Claire added two things to her night time ensemble, a blindfold and ear plugs. She was worried that she might not hear me if I needed her in the middle of the night, but she was by this time getting a little sleep deprived (actually, she was extremely sleep deprived). Between worry, travel time to the hospital, packing, unpacking, and just the business of noise and light, she had averaged about 4-5 hours sleep over the last seven nights, and for my darling wife, that wasn't even close to enough!

Day 9

When we woke up, we started to address some of our more pressing financial issues. We had planned to be gone from home for four days; it was now over a week and we had no idea when we would be able to leave. We realized that although we almost exclusively use electronic banking, we didn't know how much we owed each creditor until we got their paper bills in the mail, and some of those bills were piling up in our mailbox at home, so we made a list of those (funny how our internet service provider cannot give us e-bills), and Claire called each of our creditors, briefly explained our situation, and asked for them to send us an email with the current balance and their mailing address so that we could pay them (assuming we ever got internet access).

While Claire was busy with this, Miriam came in and we started work. The first thing that she did was get me READY for the therapy. She had brought some new fashionable clothing for me to wear, and I must admit it was a new wardrobe look. She had chosen something called TED hose, compression stockings in a lovely shade of white, which went from my toes to my groin. These were followed in the epitome of high couture, by ace bandages, two on each leg, no less, wrapped tightly from my ankle to my groin, and this was complemented by an abdominal binder, wrapped around my tummy, all in an effort to keep my blood up near my head! I just hoped Claire wouldn't take a photograph and post it to Facebook.

Once I was dressed to her satisfaction she got me up on the side of the bed and checked my blood pressure. It dropped. My blood pressure control system had not gotten the message and it was not yet ready to come out and play, and my heart rate was elevated as it was working harder than normal to try and get blood moving to where it needed to be. Claire asked me how I was feeling and I told her "I feel light headed, I feel pain and I think I am going to throw up". I realized that this was probably not very helpful information, so together we invented two new scales: The "how close am I to passing out" index; and the "how close am I to throwing up" index. Both scales went from 0-10, with 0 indicating normal operation, while anything over a 5 was an alert that things were getting serious, and that if we went much longer there was a great risk that I would either a: pass out or b: hurl in your general direction. We explained these indices to both Miriam and Karen, and they became part of our ongoing regular routine: checking readings on the "Keith Meter" so that they could either take cover or tip me over when necessary.

Things were pretty busy in rehab. After OT it was time for PT. I was scheduled for four forty-five minute sessions of therapy each day, and I realized that this was why I had been visited in the hospital: To determine whether or not I was a good rehab candidate. I had to be prepared to make not just an effort, but a good effort, and in my mind I was, but my body was not quite on board. This time, when Karen came in and I sat up, I reported a "7" on my "I am about to pass out" index, but when Karen checked my blood pressure it was normal.

This was the first of several issues which proved to me that I could no longer trust the messages that were coming from my body. Of course, we didn't push it at first to see if I actually would pass out; something tells me that this wouldn't have been considered "good medical care", but we had to retrain my blood pressure monitoring system to take care of me, and that training meant that I would have to live with feeling that I was going to pass out for a few moments before they lowered me back to horizontal. It was very uncomfortable!

At noon a miracle happened! We had internet access in our room! We were thrilled, but perplexed; we couldn't figure out how or why it had happened. There were four Ethernet ports in the room, and we had tried each one with no success, but now suddenly it was working. We discovered later that the Ethernet ports had to be switched ON to connect to the server, so thanks to Claire's "intensity" and the neuropsychologist, and all the other people who had passed the message along, the IT guys had finally switched on the Ethernet ports in our room. We went crazy! We started sending emails, making Facebook updates, looking at bank account balances (and cringing, remember no work = no pay when you are self employed) and paid the bills we could. We also started what would be a long series of serious impositions on our friends!

Our neighbors Will and Laura across the street always watched over our house when we were away, and so we called them and walked them through our house so they could get all the things we needed (checkbooks, medicine, study materials, bills, etc.) Claire also called the staff at our post office and gave them a brief update on our situation, and asked if they could help by giving our mail to Will and Laura. They were terrific, and made it all easy!

During my afternoon PT I managed to stay sitting upright for several minutes without feeling light headed. Apparently, the way you train your body's blood pressure monitoring system is to push it to behave! Sit up, when you feel dizzy stay sitting up for a bit longer, and it will adjust itself. Fascinating things, our bodies! I also managed to use a board and scoot across to an electric wheelchair, and after a literal crash course in how to drive it, I was guiding it up and down the corridors like a pro! It was FUN! This was like the first real FUN I had had in all these days, and I didn't want to stop! I found the speed controller and switched it to max (I assumed, like any motor, you had to run it at maximum speed so it was most fuel efficient, even if it was an electric motor driven by a battery), but all this fun made me tired, so I went back to bed and actually sat upright at an angle of 35 degrees without feeling dizzy.

The bed I had at rehab was much better than a standard hospital bed. I could do wonderful things with it like turn it into a chair and vibrate the mattress. One of the problems with being paralyzed is that a patient can easily develop pressure sores, which if left unattended can become infected, so the modern rehab beds have features that the nurse can control to make the bed oscillate so that you are constantly moving and hence reduce the likelihood of pressure sores.

At night I was attached to shackles made of inflatable fabric which inflate and deflate with reasonably regular but annoying frequency all the time you are trying to sleep. The nurses claimed, just like my parents always did, that it was for my own good, and would help prevent DVT (Deep Vein Thrombosis) in me because I was immobile. Maybe it's true, I haven't seen the clinical studies, but I do know the things were always malfunctioning, the cords got disconnected, and the units would occasionally pick on one leg only. Whatever they did, there was one thing they didn't do. They didn't prevent me from getting burned by my laptop power supply.

Claire was helping me change my clothes when she looked down and saw a big "blob" on my right thigh. She exclaimed "What is that!" and I looked down at my right thigh and saw a blister the size of a quarter that had been caused by the power supply on my HP laptop which had gotten so hot that it actually burned my skin. Because I had no sensation in my body below my chest, I hadn't detected any pain, and suddenly I realized how careful I was going to have to be to ensure that I avoided injuries! On a side note, Claire ultimately spoke with the people at HP who said that they were very sorry, but the computer had come with a warning not to use it on my lap. Thank you very much! Do they not call them "laptops"?

The night was another rough one for both of us. There were constant interruptions, and neither of us got anywhere near enough sleep. We both realized that this arrangement wasn't going to work. Claire needs about one to two hours more sleep than I do, every day, and this was definitely not happening in rehab. At various intervals nurses would come into the room to check vital signs, do bladder scans, give medicine, and by this time I was on intermittent catheterization, so that got added into the mix.

Sleep deprivation is no picnic, and it subtly creeps up on you until before you know it, you are behaving totally irrationally. Claire realized this when one morning she started snapping at me as though we had been fighting for years! She made an instantaneous decision that her sleep was as important to my recovery as my sleep was, and that she would be no help to me at all if she wasn't taking care of herself. We knew that everything that happens in a hospital happens for a reason, but we wondered if sometimes those reasons weren't ever looked at once the policy was made.

For example, I know that doctors want the results of all the blood work in the morning when they arrive, but does that really mean that all the blood must be drawn at 5:00 am? Why not draw some the night before, thereby allowing some patients an extra two hours of sleep in the morning? I know for some blood tests, it is important that the patient be fasting, so a morning draw is important, but is that true for all patients and tests? Does taking a patient's vital signs every four hours really ensure that the patient will live for the four hours between taking vital signs? Isn't it possible, for some patients at least, to creep silently into their rooms and check visually that they are still breathing? You might even be able to do this without waking them up; thereby allowing them a bit more uninterrupted sleep!

Claire decided to become more aggressive in looking for a hotel nearby, and she mentioned this to Belinda. In less than 45 minutes Belinda came back to her with one that was quite nearby for $2,000 for 30 days, two thirds the price of anything Claire had found. Such a deal! She made a reservation sight unseen starting Monday, August 2nd, and set about figuring out how to get there.

One of our favorite nurses during the entire experience (thankfully there were many favorites) was Keenan. Keenan was a man with a plan! Among other things, he was a natural teacher/trainer, and we talked about my future, and he explained that if my urinary tract didn't regain normal function, I would have to learn to catheterize myself. It was bad enough when four times a day someone I hardly knew came in and stuck a tube in my plumbing, but to have to fold my body in half and do it alone?

Tonight was the night, he intended to teach me how to take matters into my own hands, literally, something I never imagined I would ever need to be good at. He oozed competence and serenity as he demonstrated how to open the sterile catheter kit, how to remove the extra stuff they put in every kit, just in case you need it and then showed me the trickiest part, putting on the latex gloves without touching them on the outside. For him, it was easy! For me, with my large hands, it was a real challenge. Later I would find a supply of sterile gloves large enough for my hands, but for now, it was interesting having to stretch them on without touching them anyplace except at the very bottom of the cuff. Then he demonstrated how to open the tube of Betadine and squirt it all over five little white cotton balls without getting it all over everything else. Then, he showed me how to take the tube of gel that also came in the kit, and coat the end of the frighteningly long, very red, catheter tube that was then going to be inserted in my pipe to drain my bladder. I was nervous just looking at it. It was the second time I thanked God that I had no feeling in my sensitive parts, because I knew how painful this might normally have been. In my current state it was actually not too bad. Keenan was a great teacher, and it was clear that he knew what he was doing.

After this lesson, it was my turn to try it for real. He watched as I made a complete mess of everything, the Betadine squirted all over the place, the cotton balls would not become completely soaked, but I struggled on and managed to achieve a successful bladder drain. Keenan judged that I had earned a B+ which was not bad for a first attempt.

Day 10

On arrival, during our indoctrination, we had been told that every morning by 6:00 am, a schedule for the day would be posted on my wall, so that I would know what appointments I had, and when (like I was going to be somewhere else?) Our first morning, at 7:00 am, we asked if we had a schedule because it hadn't been posted yet. Someone came back in with a schedule and posted it on the wall. The second morning, the schedule wasn't available at 6:00 am either. Hmmmm. Something about this procedure seemed to be broken. We later found out that the schedules were all made up the night before, so there was no reason we could discern that we couldn't actually have our schedules the night before, except that for some reason that wasn't a part of the procedure. As

63

planners, it was important to us to know what was happening in advance, but that wasn't a part of our therapy.

On Day 10 my first scheduled event was OT at 7:45 am. Unfortunately, my bowel program, which was supposed to start at 6:30 am, hadn't. We have sort of glossed over this, but let me mention here, that among other things since neither my bowels nor my bladder were functioning without assistance, the "fix" was intermittent catheterization to train that pesky little valve that controls the flow of urine to open and close on demand, and a bowel program to get my bowels to "move" at approximately the same time, every day. To do this required a rigorous program of regular laxatives and stool softeners, followed by early morning insertion of a suppository; digitally (yet another finger up my butt) stimulating my rectum, and then hopefully...... poop! But this day the suppository and stimulation were one hour late, so when Miriam showed up at 7:45 am, I was delayed by ...... poop, so by 8:00 in the morning I had already missed 25% of my scheduled therapy.

In planning my bowel program one of the first considerations was when my "normal" flow occurred. For me it was in the morning, so the "plan" was to replicate that as closely as possible. That was well intended, but it didn't exactly work out well. It turns out that to replicate my "normal" operations I needed to have my suppository and "digital stimulation" at 6:00 am. Apparently, this was not a good time for the nursing staff. Most members of staff were busy getting their charting done to get ready for shift change, and so my bowel program was overlooked. This would easily have been remedied if we had been told that 6:00 am was not a terrific time for them, in which case we would have said "great, let's do it at 5:30, after the blood suckers come!" Easy fix, but the bowel program just didn't happen on time! (This was not always the case. There were night nurses who managed to make it happen regardless of whatever duties they had.)

The intermittent catheterization program was also not quite sufficient. I could easily produce 700 ml every six hours, but they were only "cathing" me once per 8 hour shift, and at one point, I produced 1.3 liters, so now every six hours instead of every eight hours someone would come in grab my private part and stick a tube into my bladder. Sounds like fun, huh? I was very grateful that I had no feeling in the little guy!

One of the staff (who shall remain nameless) had told me that I would be in rehab for at least four weeks, so we started to settle in. We put our photographs on the walls; we rearranged the furniture and were becoming familiar with the menu. This was now "home."

After breakfast Claire got me dressed in my TED hose, ace bandages, abdominal binder, sweat pants and sweat shirt, and Karen helped me transfer into the electric chair (sounds weird doesn't it?) This electric chair had wheels, and hopefully wouldn't be fatal. I followed Karen and drove myself to a room that looked like a cross between a gym and a torture chamber. Karen told me that this was the activity room, and I could only imagine the kinds of activities that she was talking about. There were all kinds of restraints attached to the ceiling and the walls, and there were pieces of equipment and low flat platforms that could be used for all kinds of creative purposes. I began to wonder what kind of people became physical therapists!

Karen helped me transfer from the chair to a low platform and then she instructed me in some yoga type exercises, and as I worked at them she told me that my progress was phenomenal! It was really hard for me to equate what I was capable of with "progress", but I was not the expert here, and so if she believed that what was happening with me was phenomenal, then I was happy. (I have found out since that every Physical therapist tells every patient that their progress is phenomenal. These people, eternal optimists, "always look on the bright side of life". They must be retired cheerleaders.) I realized that I had to give up my previous concept of what was "normal". I had assumed that "normal" meant my physical condition on July 19th, but I had replaced this foolish notion with a rather ill defined concept that I was calling "The New Normal". My goal was now to make sure that there was forward momentum. I needed to work every day to do more, longer, than the day before; as for how much better and how much more? I left that to the experts. I just wouldn't quit striving to be the best that I could be, or at least an army of one!

After lunch I felt nauseous when I transferred to the chair, so I worked on staying in the wheelchair for as long as I could in an attempt to train my body to tolerate being upright. Ciara, the Recreation Therapist came by and asked me if I felt up to a "Peer Visit". Periodically patients who had been on the unit previously would come by and offer to speak with current patients about their experiences, and apparently there was one in the unit that day. We said we would be happy to meet someone, and so a few minutes later we had a visit from a young man, Dwayne, who was in a wheelchair. He introduced himself and told us his story.

A year before, he had fallen in his garage and had broken his back becoming permanently paralyzed from the waist down. He had been in the rehab unit for six weeks but had never recovered the use of his legs, and he was very frank about the kind of challenges he faced every day. Our conversation quickly turned to pee and poop, and he laughed, telling us that whenever people who are paralyzed get together, the conversation always revolves around those two subjects! It was great to see someone with a positive attitude who was capable of independence (he drove himself wherever he needed to go and assembled his own wheelchair on arrival). We were encouraged!

For the afternoon therapy session I got into my electric chair, went to the activity room, and actually stood for the first time for about 10 seconds between two sets of parallel bars. It felt really great to be vertical again, even if it was only for a brief moment. On the way back from therapy I had a chance to drive my chair outside and to breathe what passed for fresh air in a big city in northern California.

I got to show off my new found driving skills later when a co-worker from my client came by to visit. Silena coordinated all of my teaching activities, schedules, room arrangements etc., and also processed my invoices, so she was a VIP to me, and when she came to visit she also brought with her two big bags of healthy snacks for me to munch on, which was great, since I was always hungry! What a great treat to get a visit from her, so of course I had to show off my new driving skills, so she and I took a tour of the unit as I tried to impress her with my strength, ability, and energy. She, more than anyone, needed to know that I would get well and once again be able to teach. She stayed for a nice long visit, which was great, not just because Claire and I both really like her, but also because it was really wonderful to chat with someone from outside the system and outside the crisis.

Later that day Ciara came by and asked if I would like to go to the Peer meeting where I would meet another former patient who had been on the unit two years previously with TM. I agreed to go thinking that this would be very helpful, so at the appointed hour she came to get me, and after checking that my blood pressure was OK, decided that I was well enough to attend the meeting. In this case I discovered quickly that the meeting was really an opportunity for a guest speaker to talk about lobbying and agitating for increased rights and access for the disabled. I looked around at the audience, three of us all sitting in wheelchairs. Talk about preaching to the choir; we agreed with her, but the people making the decisions didn't sit in our wheelchairs, and we were obviously not sitting in the right chairs to pass legislation or to make decisions about access to public transport or buildings.

After she finished her speech I did have an opportunity to speak with the patient who had TM. His TM event had been two years earlier, but it was neither diagnosed nor treated for two months. Since then his recovery had been steady but very slow. He was still in awful pain, still paralyzed from the waist down, and he couldn't sit comfortably in his wheelchair for any length of time. He had to give up work, and he managed from day to day on a constant diet of pain medication. I found the whole encounter was depressingly sad, but it served as negative motivation. I was now determined that this would not be my future if I had any say in it!

I can be inspired by negative motivation. In school I had a problem with my physics teacher; we were in class one day sitting on the benches watching him demonstrate an experiment, and I accidentally kicked over a stool. He glared at me and said "Launchbury, why did that stool fall over?" I replied "Sir, because the center of gravity was displaced from the point of balance, and the resulting moment of inertia created an inevitable downward path". He said "See me after class", and after class he informed me that I would never be any good in physics. I intended to prove him wrong and later went on to graduate with a degree in applied physics! I always wanted to go back and say to him, "See, I did do well," but he would have probably only remembered me as a smart aleck trouble maker.

During the day I was generally too busy to catheterize myself, it took much longer when I did it, but that evening I did my midnight "cath" under the supervision of my night nurse, and she gave me an A+!

Day 11

I was now pre-medicating with a blood pressure medicine before each therapy session. The medicine of choice was Midodrine which increases blood pressure, and it worked well and my blood pressure remained stable. During one session Miriam took me to the transitional suite where patients and their partners get to experiment with independent living before they go home. It is an efficiency apartment with a queen sized bed, a stove, refrigerator, cabinets and a sink, as well as a table and chairs. In the suite I transferred from my wheelchair to the bed, did some exercises and was able to get up and back into my chair without any support rails.

When I came back to my room I felt so confident that I decided that I could transfer on my own to the commode chair in my bathroom. As I did my knees buckled beneath me, and I sank down to the floor. Luckily, because my arms could support my weight, I didn't fall, but I had some difficulty getting back up because of the weakness in my legs. Claire was distraught! She couldn't lift me, but she managed to help me to get up enough to swing myself back into the wheelchair and to get back to bed, after which she explained to me that I had to wait until I was taught how to do something before I attempted it.

Unfortunately, this wasn't the last time I attempted to do something beyond my capabilities without training, but that seems to be how I learn best – trial and error or trial and success! Either way, I learn!

Karen wasn't available, so I had a male physical therapist, Greg, who took me to the torture chamber (activity room) where I tried to stand again but was unsuccessful. Greg was a physical therapist/sadist who really bought into this whole "pain is weakness leaving the body" nonsense. In my case, I was feeling no pain but I still had plenty of weakness that wasn't going anywhere. I am more into the "pain happens, deal with it, and try to avoid narcotics unless everything else has failed" theory, but even that wasn't applicable to me.

He must have been a marine drill instructor in a previous life but had probably quit because it was too easy for him. He sure knew how to push me around! He had me dancing to his tune doing tough exercises and pushing myself to my absolute maximum limit, which I am sure was good for me, but was taxing and exhausting! When I was unsuccessful doing things vertically, he pushed me to do some new things horizontally, and when our 45 minutes were over, I was relieved and exhausted!

When Miriam came back for OT Claire told her about my commode chair experiment, so Miriam taught me how to use the commode chair correctly! First it had to be set at the right height, then one of the arms had to be lowered, and then I could transfer. Finally Miriam gave me a gift beyond compare! She told me that she would teach me how to take a shower by myself! Up to this point, we were still doing bed baths and rinse free shampoo, and it felt just terrific to have my first real shower. I had nearly forgotten what "normal" was. For me, normal was to get up, work out for 90 minutes or so, shower, and attack the day. None of that was in my schedule now, so when I had my first shower, it was like a light at the end of the tunnel was suddenly, though dimly, visible. I realized that the more closely things matched what was usual at home, the less stress there would be for me, so things like taking showers in the morning were really great!

After lunch it was PT with Greg again, but this time he brought in a tilt table. A tilt table is basically a flat platform that can rotate 90 degrees, from horizontal to vertical. The patient can be belted in, and then be raised to an upright position to allow weight on his/her feet and legs. I thought it would be great to see if I could "feel" my legs underneath me, since I had no sensation in them, and I wanted to see if I could stand upright without my blood pressure tanking. Greg strapped me to the bed and slowly raised it up to an almost vertical position. I stood upright normally for ten minutes, thrilled beyond belief as my blood pressure remained steady, and I remained "0-0" on my indices. I was so proud of myself; I could actually feel my legs beneath me and it felt really good. Claire took pictures, and after therapy Claire took me and my wheelchair for a walk outside the hospital to enjoy some of the beautiful weather.

Despite the successes, we were unbelievably stressed since we had no idea how much recovery we could expect, and yet every day we were more and more encouraged, as I gained more control, more strength, and more ability. Each night before bed we prayed for God to continue to grant me additional healing and we knew that our friends, our church family, and our biological family were all adding their prayers to ours. Every day we could report new progress and new improvement on Facebook and every day we got back incredible messages of support from around the world. The photographs of me on the tilt table were the first we took, and hindsight being 20/20, I wish that we had taken photos earlier so that we could have something to compare them to as we went along. The reality was, however, that no one wants to have their photos taken when at their worst, and until this point I was pretty badly off, and photos of a grown man in a hospital gown lying flat on his back do not make for encouraging images.

Chapter 4 - In Crisis

Day 12

The next day when I woke up I knew immediately that something was seriously wrong. As I started trying to dress myself I realized that I had far less flexibility and mobility than the day before. We immediately called the nurse, Jane, and she responded quickly by calling Doctor Matthews who ordered an urgent MRI. I was prepped with all the required medication, oxygen and ice bag, an IV was inserted in my arm, and I was ready to be taken down to the MRI department. In some respects the MRI went well this time; they did two passes, once without and once with contrast, but there was a downside this time. In addition to being bombarded by noise, and constrained within this very confined space, I had a bowel movement halfway through the procedure. Boy was that fun! Forget about the dignity (or rather, indignity) and embarrassment, I also got to experience the full aromatic effect until the clanking was all done and I was taken back to my room and cleaned up.

Dr. Matthews was waiting for me, and he immediately put me back on IV steroids and called for backup from two neurologists, my original neurologist, Dr. Thomas, who did the diagnosis, and a new one, Dr. Graham, who was local. They all reviewed the MRI and decided, after much deliberation, to transfer me to the Intensive Care Unit at another hospital, one that was a part of the same network, but was physically located a couple of miles away, for a procedure called plasmapheresis.

Since TM is a disorder that has your own personal immune system attacking your spinal cord, the "fix" is to first: reduce the swelling of the lesions that the disorder causes, and second: to stop the immune system from attacking your body. The corticosteroids would do both, but if they didn't do enough, then the antibodies had to be removed from your body. That is what plasmapheresis does. Your blood is removed, filtered to remove the plasma which contains the antibodies, and then put back in your body. The volume that is lost through the filtering system is replaced with Albumin (a human body product like egg white, produced as a protein from the liver, but also conveniently available in a big bottle from the pharmacy). It is a bit like kidney dialysis.

Once again, our lives were being shattered by something over which we had no control. It was obvious that something was seriously wrong. I had been doing so well, and the way everyone was acting was terrifying Claire. She could see me going backwards, losing all that I had gained, and becoming totally paralyzed once again. We were all alone, so far from home, family, and friends.

Jane came in as I was getting ready to leave and I noticed that she had tears in her eyes. When I asked her what was going on, she said "You are really sick!" This, I knew, was not a good thing, but I told her "Don't worry I'll be back!" We didn't know what was going on, we knew that people were worried, but no one would tell us what was wrong.

Claire and I suddenly realized that with my transfer, she, four suitcases, and four carry-on bags were suddenly homeless! So, to add to her overwhelming worry about me, she had to once again pack up four suitcases and four carry-on bags and get them someplace by herself. She was overwhelmed by the task, severely stressed by the crisis, and could have used a calm presence as well as some packing assistance.

As I have mentioned, we are very spiritual people, so when I was asked on admission if I was interested in being visited by a minister from a local church, I said that I was! Somehow, that never happened. I would have really appreciated a visit, someone besides Claire to listen to my thoughts as I tried to see God's plan in what was happening to me and someone who could help me find more positive aspects of our journey to focus on than those we had found ourselves. I know that as a part of most admission procedures, patients are asked about religious preferences, and if they would like a visit, but I have no idea what happened with that information. Had we been in our local hospital, our pastor would have been there like a shot, but we were strangers in a strange land, and since we were hardly ever in California on Sundays, we didn't have a local church home so we didn't have anyone to contact.

Thankfully, Claire was able to get a room two days earlier than she had planned at the nearby hotel, and she was able to reach Mark, the student who had visited us with his chocolates. Mark came to the rehab unit and took two of the suitcases home with him, took her to check in at the hotel, and brought her to the hospital! You would have thought that she had just gotten a reprieve from a death sentence. Everything was magnified. If it was bad, it was torturous, and if it was good, it was exhilarating. What a blessing he was to her, and to me, since I didn't have to worry about her, and could concentrate on what was happening to me!

Being rushed to the Intensive Care Unit of any Hospital is never a good thing, and I had a lot of time to reflect while I waited to be transported by ambulance. I was imagining all the things that could be wrong with me, that would have caused the doctors at Rehab to push the panic button and transfer me to ICU. No one told me what was going on, what was wrong, and what was going to be done. All I knew was that they were transferring me to an ICU, and in my experience, anyone in an ICU was in serious trouble.

I had to deal with the fact that I might be really sick and might lose all the ground that I had gained, all the movement I had become capable of, and all the independence I had mastered. I mentally checked off all my functions: I wasn't in any pain, my lungs appeared to be operating normally, I still had strength in my upper body, I was not about to pass out, and my legs still had some mobility, although far less than previously, but I was still on my way to the ICU. My brain appeared to be functioning as well as it ever had, not that you could have ever called it normal! My basic life support systems appeared to be running quite well on automatic, so it wasn't all bad, so I had to deal with the prospect that there was something seriously wrong me that I couldn't define. I asked myself if I was ready to give up this life and move on to whatever comes next.

I have always been a Christian, though recently I have found my faith has become deeper and stronger than at any time in my life. As a small child in England my parents took me to church, and as a bigger child they sent me to church, but when I became a teenager I was very keen to go to church. In our small village it was the only place outside of school where we could meet people our own age, and our minister had two attractive teenage daughters, so quite a few of the young men in our village became churchgoers, keen on singing in the choir and ringing bells, joining the youth group and doing lots of other church related activities. We had great fun and I especially remember the church outings, the sponsored walks for charity, and the all night walks to discover the beauty of God's creation and try to get close to the minister's daughters.

Over the years I had gone to church, at first, when obliged, then by habit, and occasionally I got something spiritual from the process, but since I had met my wife I had truly become a more committed Christian. She reinforced my belief in the healing and redemptive power of Jesus Christ. I had witnessed miracles. I had felt God's love and presence in my life. I read the Bible on a regular basis; I worked in the church, went on mission trips and truly believed that God was close by, so I knew that God was with me. It was easy to tell Jane that I would be back; I had faith that it would be so.

When I lost control of my body I recognized the reality that we are never really in control. I had been deluding myself for most of my life by telling myself that I was running my own business, making my own decisions, and living my own life, and I liked the feeling that I was in control. Now it was obvious that I was not in control, so now I had to start again, let go and let God take over. I wasn't giving up; I was prepared to do whatever I could, and to accept whatever kind of life that God was prepared to give me. I believe that Jesus had healed the sick and made the lame walk, and I had the additional benefit of 2000 years of medical advancement. I would not have to be carried by my friends and put in the middle of a busy street to beg for food. I had a lot going for me!

In February I had bought long term care insurance and now it seemed amazing that I might actually get the benefit of the program after paying only one premium! I had excellent health insurance (thanks to my wife and her 20 years of military service) and Claire had shown me how much she loved me in health, and now had her chance to show me how much she loved me in sickness.

My wife is a much better caregiver than she is a patient, which was proven when she broke her rib a couple of years previously. It was all "just leave me alone until I ask you for something" and me feeling helpless. I am the opposite. We had talked about how really glad we both were that this had happened to me, and not to her. We were both far better equipped to deal with it this way around. My job was to get well, and I had the discipline and strength to do it. Her job was to ensure that the environment was conducive to my recovery, and she sure had the training and personality for that, so I knew what I had to do, I knew the awesome power of God, and I had unshakeable faith in Claire. I had a positive attitude, I believed in the power of prayer. I felt the presence of God in my life so I didn't dwell on the past and I accepted my future. While waiting for the ambulance I had a conversation with God that went something like this:

OK God, you have my attention; you are in control, not me.
I know I have been fooling myself all these years, but now I truly understand.
I am paralyzed and 60% of my body doesn't work right.
I accept that you are in charge, and I would really like it if you could restore some of my basic systems, but I will accept whatever you give me.
Thanks for letting my brain still work.
I sure would like to walk again, if that would be OK with you.
It would be nice if I did not have to live with constant pain.
My wife would be really happy if I could have bowel and bladder control as well.
The rest we can live with. Thank you.

The reality was that I was attempting to bargain with God, but I knew that He was ultimately in control, directing my life, giving me my purpose, and I knew that He would grant me strength and show me what I needed to do. When you know this, you can truly be at peace.

This was the first time in my life that I had ever been in an Intensive Care Unit, and it was not fun. The first thing that they do is stick things all over your body so that they can hook up wires and monitor you every minute of the day and night. They connect these wires to displays and monitors which make noises when things go wrong and attract your attention like those annoyingly loud television sets that are installed in too many medical waiting rooms. You don't want to watch them and you can't change the channel but they prevent you from quiet relaxation, calm conversations, or reading a book. You end up yelling like people in a noisy bar.

The other aspect of life in an ICU is that there is no day or night; there is always activity and noise. Most patients are too sick to care about this, but I wasn't. The ICU is where only the sickest patients are sent. Tell someone you are going to the ICU and they start thinking morbid thoughts, and my mother, my children, my grandchildren and my friends, thousands of miles away, were extremely worried.

Another thing that became obvious really quickly was that the other patients in the ICU were much worse off than I was. I know it was quite a novelty for the staff to be bringing someone food on a tray, someone who could hold a fork, and carry on a conversation over dinner. My next door neighbor was clearly confused. He didn't know where he was, he didn't speak English, and he spent most of his time screaming and yelling for help. I spoke to the nurses about this, and suggested several helpful ways in which this could be more pleasant. Valium, sleeping pills and duct tape were all suggested, but the nursing staff told me that they were not options. My next suggestion was noise reduction headphones and IPods. The nurse agreed that it was a good idea and said that he would bring it up at the next management meeting, but somehow I got the feeling that I would not be getting any help in the short term, so I used my own MP3 player, put in my own headphones and turned my music on loud. This instantly drowned out the screamer next door, but also made it difficult for the nursing staff to get my attention.

I was working on inventing a device that they could use when they needed to talk to me, based on the same idea as the telephone headset for the deaf that I saw demonstrated in a Monty Python episode: A deaf person wore a headset with a big red light that would flash when the phone rang, then they could answer the phone. One bad point, unfortunately, being deaf they still couldn't hear the person on the other end of the phone line. I was still working out the bugs in my design when I realized it was futile; I was fighting a losing battle. In order to drown out the screamer, I had to turn my music up so loud that I couldn't rest or sleep, but if I had it on quietly, then the screams for help would keep me awake. I realized that the other guests in ICU were on such heavy drugs that they didn't care. I was on my own in unchartered territory, I had lost my guide and my GPS couldn't find any satellites. I had just started trying to figure out when I could get some sleep when a young girl about our daughter's age walked in to my room, smiled at me and said, "Hi I'm Kaitlyn and I am your doctor".

It was clear to me that any idea I had of healthcare in America had gone straight out the window. She didn't look like any doctor I had ever seen in my life, and I felt really old! Kaitlyn had read my chart, she knew my history and what was more, she was particularly interested in me because she wanted to be a neurologist, and after all, how often do you come across transverse myelitis cases! I was going to be her first "interesting patient."

She told me the plan. She was going to insert a large diameter vascular catheter in my jugular vein. That sure didn't sound good to me, so I asked her "Why?", and she explained that it was necessary for the plasmapheresis treatments that my neurologist had ordered for me. I reminded her that 60% of my body could feel no pain, but that the 60% didn't include my neck, so I asked her if there wasn't some other place that they could put in this catheter, but she told me she needed a large vein and there were only three places that she could use:-

- My groin (not my first choice!);
- My thigh (that would be fine with me since I couldn't feel that), and
- My neck (the location of choice for medical professionals).

It seems that the groin and thigh are too likely to become contaminated, and you don't want any contamination when you take bodily fluids out, mess around with them, and put them back in, so it was decided that I would get a jugular catheter. I hated to ask her if she had ever done one before, but I assumed she had spent her childhood doing science experiments on pet animals so it was probably going to be OK.

The procedure involved me looking the other way and holding my head still as she stuck a pipe the size of a fire hydrant in my neck. "Don't move" she said "or I might sever your carotid artery by accident." This didn't sound like a good thing; I didn't remember much from my biology lessons in school, but I vaguely remember that severed arteries are a bloody nuisance, so I was sufficiently afraid that I remained still and let her finish the procedure. When she was done I felt proud of my one sided necklace of dangling tubes and I couldn't wait to show people, but then she covered it up with bandages and adhesive tape because it wasn't needed just then.

Day 13

My screamer next door screamed all night long, but then he was quiet during the day, but it didn't matter, there was no way anyone would let me sleep in the daytime. People kept coming by. They came to stick needles in my veins, draw blood, hook me up to IV's, take my blood pressure, take my temperature, doctors came in to ask questions, check my lungs, see if I had any reflexes, do rectal examinations, nurses came in to do catheterizations, clean up my mess, bring my food, and then there were the inevitable problems with the equipment. "I think one of your leads is off." "I don't think we are picking you up." "I think the battery is gone in the unit", etc., etc., etc. This never happened on Star Trek! The Doctor would come in with a medical tricorder and know everything about you. With all the zillions of dollars we spend on health care you would think someone would have come up with one by now. So you can't sleep at night and you can't rest by day. If you weren't sick in the first place, you would be soon!

I realized that what my Great Aunt Vera had told me was true. I asked her on her 100th birthday what the secret was to a long life, and she reflected over her whole career in nursing, and gave me two great pieces of advice: "Avoid doctors and never go to the hospital." It was true; so like a prisoner of war, I started to formulate my escape plan. I would not stay in the ICU, I didn't belong there. I was all set to start ripping off the leads, and make a run for the door, when I realized that I still couldn't walk.

Then, as if that wasn't enough, they also wanted a tube in my arm. They wanted the ability to hook me up to an IV very quickly, so they looked at my arms and decided that they should insert a couple of extra IV lines there "just in case". Apparently, when you are in a hospital you can never have too many tubes stuck into your body, and so every patient gets a couple of needles attached to tubes stuck in their veins, and these have to be changed every four days, so then they get to do it all over again.

When I was young I was very squeamish, I fainted at the sight of blood, especially if it was mine! Since I had grown up I had somewhat overcome this phobia (although Claire did have to be the one to go in the room when the plastic surgeon was sewing up our daughter after a car accident) and I have even become a regular blood donor, so I was used to people sticking needles in my veins, but now I felt like a pin cushion. People were doing it on purpose; they had deliberately chosen areas of my body where I could feel pain, and they were blithely ignoring the places where I wouldn't feel a thing. It was so unfair!

In the evening my new neurologist, Dr. Graham, came in to visit, and he explained why I had been transferred so quickly to the ICU. He actually spent over an hour with us, and answered every question we had in depth and with detail. It was a huge relief to be able to understand what was happening and why! Dr. Graham explained that the original MRI on July 21st (day 2) had shown lesions on my spinal column from T5-T9 and T11 - T12, but the MRI on July 31st (day 12) showed lesions on ALL the thoracic vertebrae from T1-T12. This had escalated the magnitude and extent of the transverse myelitis, and now I had Longitudinally Extensive Transverse Myelitis (LETM) which was considerably worse.

This caused grave concern because there was a widely held view that LETM was caused by Neuro Myelitis Optica (NMO) which most probably would lead to blindness. Dr. Graham also explained that while a TM attack does most of its damage in the first 24-48 hours, it can keep causing damage for up to 21 days after the initial attack. He hoped to start me on plasmapheresis to remove antibodies from my blood as soon as possible and he planned to send samples of my blood and spinal fluid (great, another spinal tap) to the Mayo clinic so that they could test for the NMO marker.

As it happens we discovered later that there was an error on the MRI report. The MRI report said that there was involvement of the C5-C6 vertebrae, but two days later the MRI report was amended to reflect that there had been a typo in the original report, and there was no involvement of the cerebral vertebrae. It reminded Claire of why the Navy used a phonetic alphabet – to avoid confusion. While C5 might sound like T5, Charlie is never going to sound like Tango. The amendment meant that there was no involvement on T1-T4.

There is a web based support group for people with TM, and I received a message from someone with TM who asked me about my treatment and recovery. Kristine told me that when she asked her own neurologist which vertebrae were impacted by her own TM, he told her "You don't need to know that". I was glad that Dr. Graham had leveled with me and told me the truth, because now I could deal with it, share the information with my family and friends, and now we had specific things to ask God for.

After a full night and day in the ICU, this terrific information, and a complete lack of real rest, I was ready to attempt to try to get some real sleep. I spoke with my nurse and she told me that the doctors wanted to do a spinal tap, but they were talking about waiting until the morning, and she was glad, because even she knew that I needed my rest. She lowered the lights and closed the door. I thanked her very much, plugged my earphones in my ears, turned on my MP3 player and fell into a sound sleep. An hour later I was woken from my sleep by four doctors in my room telling me that they were going to do a spinal tap; this was a teaching hospital, and tonight I was the subject. They had selected me as their guinea pig, and they would all have a go at a lumbar puncture; "after all he can't feel it, so he is perfect". The first doctor tried to do the spinal tap but couldn't get the needle in the right place. After about ten minutes of trying, the second doctor took over, with equally unsuccessful results. The senior doctor kept giving advice, but nothing worked. A third doctor tried and failed as well, so at this point the expert took over and said "This is how you do it, and it is a good thing he can't feel what is going on." She tried and she failed as well. After one hour of sticking needles into my back, they all decided to call it quits, and said "Why don't you go back to sleep, we will ask the radiologist to do it in the morning." I hoped that I had been dreaming, but the nurse confirmed later that she had tried to keep them out, but the doctors call the shots in the hospital in every sense of the word, and I got her point. I can't think of any reason other than an emergency that would require the disruption of a patient's sleep to give four doctors the chance to try their hand at a spinal tap. It simply could have been just as easily and readily earlier in the day when I was awake, or the following morning.

Day 14

The next morning the radiologist did the spinal tap, first time, no problem, in a very simple procedure. He had the benefit of the right equipment, and it was pinpoint accurate. My nurse had told me that to avoid a headache I had to remain flat on my back for six hours following the spinal tap, and Dr. Kaitlyn (I still cannot get used to the idea of calling doctors by their first name!) came around afterwards with a cup of hazelnut coffee from the doctors' lounge, which she told me, would also help me avoid the headache that often comes after a spinal tap. It tasted great, and it worked! This time, I had no headache!

Chapter 5 - In Transition

In "The Spirit Catches You and You Fall Down" by Anne Fadiman there is an argument between two health care professionals which goes like this:

"'Which is more important, the life or the soul?'
'I make no apology,' said Bill. 'The life comes first.'
'The soul,' said Sukey."

We believe that both are critical to a patient's health and that part of the healthcare providers' jobs is to care for the soul as well as the life, but the more care you require, the less the system cares about your soul, so intensive care becomes insensitive care very quickly. There is no day or night, the lights are always on, there is always noise, people are always coming and going and every patient is at risk, so the staff does whatever is required to keep them alive, and that is the right thing! People will never complain if you save their lives! Hardly any of the patients are stable or conscious enough to know whether it is day or night, or if the nurses joke or talk about their personal business while they work. The patients just try to get well.

Time becomes irrelevant; people come and go on their schedules and as a patient, your job is to try to adapt. I just wasn't that kind of a patient, and I was afraid that I would be stuck in the ICU for an eternity! I kept hoping that they would need my bed for a more deserving (sicker patient), but unfortunately they couldn't find one. I needed to get out of there, so I was ready to grasp any lifeline that I could find.

Day 14

My first visitors following my spinal tap came around 10:00 am, when a doctor I hadn't seen before (Dr. White), surrounded by a bunch of medical people (what is the collective term for doctors? Gaggle? Docket? Drove? Doctrine?) knocked on the door, opened it and politely asked "May we come in?" as if I had any choice in the matter. She told us that these were interns and residents, and that this was "rounds." "Rounds" is when all the doctors swarm into a patient's room to talk to each other about the patient. The patient is merely an observer to the process. I suspected that the greater the number of doctors in my room at any one time, the greater the bill sent to my insurance company!

We did the same thing when I worked in a consulting firm; the managing partner had to have a weekly meeting with me about the account I was working on and after I gave him an in-depth status report, he gave me a bill for services rendered, which of course, got passed on to the client.

In the case of the doctors on rounds they can be accompanied by a case manager, a couple of hospital administrators, the unit charge nurse, your own nurse, a nursing assistant, the guy who delivers meal trays, and anyone else who is standing around with nothing to do. I looked around the tiny space that they had given me, and told her that they were welcome, but there was only room for one at a time! The doctor did smile, and they all walked in and crowded around the bottom of my bed. I could see Dr. Kaitlyn, the only friendly face I could recognize in the group, but this was after all, a teaching hospital and I was one of their science experiments, and she, one of the students. Eventually we got to know all the doctors, but when they came in for the first time for "rounds" and they were all new to us, we felt as though we were objects of unimportance, not worth of recognition or of conversation. We wanted to know who was "on first", so we would know who to call in the event we had a question, and it was always our job to find it out rather than their job to tell us.

Dr. White told them that I had Acute Transverse Myelitis (I was glad I had a cute something), and that they would not often see a case like mine. She proceeded to take out a safety pin and poke me in the foot with it. "See he doesn't react to that! He cannot detect pain below the mid thoracic vertebrae." They were talking about me, as if I wasn't there. She acted as if she could only see the "case", not the "person" and was concerned about the teaching moment rather than the healing. She went on showing them the impact of this "classic" case of TM. I wouldn't have minded if she had been talking to me, but she was talking about me to people I hadn't even been introduced to.

There may be a lot of conversations, particularly in a teaching hospital, that the patient doesn't need to participate in, and in that case, they should be held in a conference room or outside the patient's room, but when the staff are discussing the patient in the patient's room, then the conversation should be personal, and the patient and the patient's family should be engaged in it and a part of it. There is no one with a more vested interest in what is happening with the patient than the patient, and secondarily, the patient's family. To discuss the patient within their hearing, and not involve them in the conversation is not only rude and insulting, but it also overlooks the greatest source of information about the patient available, the patient and his/her family.

My mother taught me never to say anything to people unless you had been formally introduced (unlike my wife, who will start up a personal conversation with anyone), so I decided to make my presence known, and started interjecting my own "truth" in between her sentences. I believed that I was a very important part of the recovery team since I had a personal vested interest in getting well, and I wanted to make sure they all knew that I was a participant, not an object of curiosity.

They just looked quizzically at me; I guess at this point they decided that they had seen enough for the day, and moved on to more compliant patients. School was over as far as I was concerned. They had already exceeded the maximum occupancy sign that I had made for the room, and I didn't want the door to hit them as they left, but of course I couldn't get up to see them out. The group managed to find a way to let themselves out safely and so my wife and I went back to getting on with our day.

Then "help" showed up in the form of a physical therapist, Marilyn, who did an evaluation and promised that she would put me on a schedule for physical therapy every day, though she was somewhat limited by the constraints of the ICU. She also gave me some therabands which I could use to do some exercises in bed every day. These are wide rubber bands that are used to provide resistance, and can be used for a good number of exercises. I thought these particular bands were some kind of joke as they didn't offer me much resistance and I kept thinking that they would break! The other problem I had with them was when I wrapped them around my hands to hold them, they acted like a tourniquet and cut off my blood circulation. I did however, assess their possible use as a potential strangulation weapon in case I was set upon by a deranged nurse or patient.

Marilyn started me off with a yellow one, which I almost broke, followed by an orange one which was only slightly better. Then I got to try the green one and then finally a blue one, each one with increasingly higher resistance. Then Marilyn suggested that I use some of them together. I asked when I could work up to the black belt, but she informed me that purple was the highest level that they had. I admit that I was annoyed that she was concentrating on my upper body strength, which I thought was just fine, but in hindsight I realize that I was so focused on wanting to walk, that I didn't take seriously the need to keep my upper body strong.

I finally got a purple band, but even the strongest one that they had was still too little resistance for me. I thought that I was probably unusual as a patient, since I actually felt fine, but we were determined and resourceful, so when the therabands proved insufficient, Claire went out to a sporting goods store and purchased something with more resistance, so that I could feel that I was actually doing something for myself.

After the limited physical therapy, I realized that it was up to me to show them that I didn't need to be there, and that I needed to be back in Rehab, where I would get the "hard" stuff. If I couldn't actually get up and walk out of the ICU, I could at least try to prove to them that I was stable enough to be moved to a place where they didn't have to give me such intensive care. As far as I knew, I was only there for plasmapheresis, and this was now my second day and I was still waiting.

I was curious how plasmapheresis worked. At 7:00 pm, a technician who introduced himself as Franklin, finally arrived, and wheeled in a machine that took up half the space in my room. As he set up the machine Claire left us to it, as she wanted to get back to her hotel before it got dark. She was still taking taxis, and though it was now only $12 a trip, she knew that she would have to find another way!

Franklin hooked up the lines to the ports in my neck, and before long my blood was being sucked out of my body, quicker than Bill Compton (True Blood) could ever imagine. In my case Franklin had a distinct advantage over Bill; because of the blood superhighway in my neck the blood was flowing like a river. I watched in fascination as my red blood streamed out of me, and as it came back in the level of the yellow liquid in the big bottles went down, and the level of the yellow "stuff" in the clear bag went up. This was, he told me, my plasma which had been filtered out of my blood. The machine was removing it from my body and collecting it, and at the same time was topping me up with some brand new Albumin.

I was curious what he intended to do with my plasma; maybe it had some resale value, but Franklin assured me that it was heading to the medical incinerator. Apparently no one needed my used plasma. I was hoping I could sell it on EBay; it might have offset a fraction of the hospital bill. Surely someone needed my antibodies?

After 2 hours Franklin had collected about 3 liters of the stuff and I did the math. A normal healthy adult has about 5 liters of blood in their body, and the process had removed about 60% of my blood volume and put it in a bag that they intended to throw in the trash. How could they be so reckless? Franklin finished up the process, disconnected me from the machine, and took my plasma away. Once that was finished, I got to settle down to try to sleep, but of course, since I was still in the ICU, a good night's sleep was unlikely!

Day 15

The highlight of the day was the arrival of our first package from our neighbors! It included our mail including some of our Netflix DVDs, as well as medicines, Claire's checkbooks, and study materials for the upcoming class which I was scheduled to teach on August the 14th, so we could actually do WORK to prepare for teaching, but here we were on August 3rd, and the likelihood of my being able to teach in 11 days seemed very slim. We had said originally that we would wait until I had been in rehab for 10 days before making a final decision about the August 14th class, but it looked pretty clear that teaching in 11 days was not going to be possible, so we made the fateful decision, and cancelled the class. It was nice to get the package though. We could see what bills we had overlooked, and now had checkbooks so that we could pay them in case there was no internet access. We found that we were actually in better shape than we had thought we would be, so that was encouraging.

Later in the day I had a visit from Dr. Hawkins, the immunologist, who took the time to explain the science behind the plasmapheresis process. He was a great teacher; he knew his subject and he seemed to enjoy explaining it. He told me that we would repeat the procedure every other day which would allow my body some time to rebuild its own blood and plasma supply. I asked how many treatments he thought I would need, and he said that usually they scheduled between five and seven, but that there was no magic number; it really depended on the individual. He explained that if the treatments were working, then I would notice continued recovery on a daily basis; then at some point the recovery would level out and the treatments could cease. That meant a minimum of 10 days in the hospital, and potentially as long as two weeks. There was no question that the decision to cancel the August 14th class was the right one.

When we found out that the plasmapheresis was going to be done every two days, we didn't realize what that meant for my recovery, or lack thereof! I had TM and I needed plasmapheresis, but otherwise, I felt normal! For us, this meant that out of every 48 hours, 46 were wasted in terms of my recovery. As it happens, we eventually found out that the plasmapheresis could have been done at the original rehab hospital, which would have been far better for everyone, except of course the contract company doing the plasmapheresis as it was somewhat inconvenient for them to go to the other hospital when all their equipment was at this hospital, but it would have been possible, and I wouldn't have missed out on all those days of twice a day PT and twice a day OT.

Claire decided to ask the physical therapist what we could do on our own, between sessions, and she watched everything the therapist did. Then when we were on our own, she coached me through my own PT sessions. As a result, I got nearly 3 hours a day of exercise, even when nothing was scheduled for me.

Following Dr. Hawkins' visit I met Susan, a physical therapist who was great friends with Karen, the physical therapist from rehab. She did a brief evaluation since this was the first time that she had seen me, and I could honestly tell her that I felt that I was getting stronger. She was appropriately complimentary when she could see what I could do, and we gave her permission to talk with Karen about my status, since we were certain that we would soon be back in Karen's loving care! It appeared that the plasmapheresis was working. I was also seriously excited, even highly enthusiastic, when they came to tell me that my wish had been granted, and I was being transferred to a Transitional Intensive Care Unit (TICU). I would still be monitored, but the benefit of this unit was that they had remote telemetric units that could be used to monitor my vital signs from the safety of some secure location. It didn't take Claire long to pack up all my things, by this time most of it was gone from the hospital, and she was also a packing pro, and so we were ready for the move.

When I arrived at the new unit, my new medical team came by to introduce themselves. I had three interns (all female and all looked younger than our daughter) and one hospitalist (also female but older, she must have been at least 30!) on my case in addition to Dr. Kaitlyn. We immediately started calling them "The Dream Team", and they proved to be just that. My nurses, on the other hand, while highly competent, were older, mostly male and not so cute; so much for typical stereotypes.

The TICU was a step down from the ICU and it looked and felt more like a normal ward, and I was able to sleep a good five hours as it was far quieter than the ICU. I could actually play my music at a normal level and I quickly decided that I could get used to this.

My nurse came in with a cath kit (that package wrapped in white paper containing all of the necessary requirements to catheterize a patient to drain his/her bladder) and he was quite surprised when my output exceeded his one liter container, so I offered to pinch the pipe and hold it closed while he went to fetch a back up container. We executed this plan, and when I released the temporary valve I produced another 325ml. He told me that this was excessive, and he would put me on a six hour catheter program to empty my bladder more often, so I would be catheterized at six o'clock and twelve o'clock, am and pm.

We called our daughter to let her know I had been transferred to the TICU and her four year old son wanted to speak to his "Bampa". He talked with me for a minute, and then, puzzled, he asked "Bampa, how come I can't see you?" I realized that his generation is growing up in a world that is very different from the one I grew up in. He had been taught by experience to expect to see the people he was talking to, so I explained that we were using old technology, a telephone instead of a computer, and we would "see" each other again soon. He managed to carry on quite a good conversation, but he was clearly disappointed by the limitations of the telephone, highlighting for us how important that internet connection was not just to us, but to our entire family.

In the meantime, since Claire didn't have a car, she was either destined to use taxi cabs, rent a car, or find her way by public transport. A woman at the information desk took some time to teach her how to use the San Francisco Transit Authority website to figure out how to get around town by bus, which she soon did like an expert. She could get nearly anywhere! It was just a matter of taking time.

Day 16

During the night I had a dream that I was not in a wheelchair and that I was walking on my own without any assistance, and when I woke I picked up my phone and had a text message from my oldest granddaughter (age 11) asking me how I was doing. I told her about my dream of walking again, and she said "That's good, God was talking to you, and He gave you a vision". I was so impressed by her strong faith, and as it happened, she was absolutely right!

Like Scrooge, I was then visited by three ghosts; the first was the ghost of the living dead, namely an amiable lab technician who came to take my blood. He chatted casually as he stuck yet another needle into my arm, and he looked like he would fit right in with the night shift at a much hated but often visited super discount chain. I had seen their night shift, and they were definitely not always people you would look forward to seeing out during the day. I spoke with one cashier who actually admitted that she had to be in bed before the sun rose, and that made we wish that I had bought the anti vampire kit in aisle 4.

My guy from the lab looked as though he didn't just draw blood, but that he actually *needed* it. He had more tattoos than bike week at Daytona, and probably more piercings than any of Jack the Ripper's victims. He seemed happy enough, despite the early hour, and seemed to enjoy his work.

Every morning I would be awakened by someone coming in to draw blood for some tests or other. We were never told what I was being tested for, and never told what the results were. I assumed perhaps naively, that were there something worth reporting, we would hear about it, and we had so much of importance that we were obsessing about we didn't have a lot of capacity to worry about a non-issue, but it would have been really great to hear what the tests were for, and what the results were.

This was followed by a bustle of activity around the shift change and then the second ghost, the ghost of what doctors will be. One of the Dream Team came in and went through what was now a standard process. She used the stethoscope and asked me to take deep breaths and she listened to my lungs and heart ensuring no pneumonia or lung complications, she looked into my eyes to ensure that my pupils were dilating they way they should be (we joked that she had to keep an eye on my pupils just as I did when I was teaching), she asked me about whether or not I noticed any vision changes, and then she asked me to stick out my tongue and say "aaah". She then took a sharp object, and started poking me with it starting at my toes and asking me to tell her when it felt sharp. That usually occurred up around my rib cage, so she dutifully made note of this. She then put her hand on my knee asked me to raise my knee and push up against her hand with it, then the other; to push down on her hands with my feet, to curl my toes up against her hands, and to squeeze her fingers, until she realized that my upper body wasn't impacted, and I could crush them. She asked me to shrug my shoulders against her hands, push up with my elbows against her arms, push her away from me (usually her feet slid across the floor) and then pull her towards me, at which point she nearly fell into my bed, and let go giggling.

She and all the other doctors who would do this daily, were checking to make sure that I was not losing any upper body strength and that I was gaining lower body strength. I was assured that all these activities were necessary every day and they told me to let them know the moment I saw anything that looked red when it shouldn't be, as this would be a sure sign that Neuro Myelitis Optica (NMO) was in my future. The test results wouldn't come back for at least ten days, so we prayed a game of wait and see: If I could see, I could wait, and if we all prayed then perhaps the test results from the "Mayo" clinic would come back negative. I told one doctor that I wanted the samples to go to the "Miracle Whip" clinic, and she laughed. I maintained my warped sense of humor!

After the doctor's visit it was the ghost of nursing chance, my morning medication. Each pill was hermetically sealed in its own little nurse proof bubble packaging, and delivered, often separately, in its own plastic disposable container. I was mystified that they didn't reuse these cups, and I suggested it several times, but no one seemed particularly interested. I suspected that after being taken out of the trash by a guy up the street, these little cups had a quick trip through a sterilizer, and were resold to the hospital for fun and profit.

As an expert in the field of Supply Chain Management I was appalled by the level of waste in the medical supply chain. No wonder health care costs are out of control. There was so much potential for more efficient management of the hospital supply chain. I fully understand the need to minimize the risk of potential contamination between patients, so everything has to be thrown away, but it seems to me the pendulum has swung too far in favor or risk mitigation, and that the level of waste and duplication is excessive. I believe that pretty soon hospitals will be spending more money on their supply chain then they do in paying their service providers. I just want to get well enough to help solve these problems and start addressing the very real issues of reducing costs through improved Supply Chain Management.

I never knew what to expect when a nurse walked in with my medication. Every nurse was supposed to check my wrist band and my name, and take the time to tell me the medication I was receiving and give me the reason why the medication was being given. Some nurses did a very good job, some were OK, but others were bad. Human errors were made, and my wife and I caught as many as we could, but we were never assured that some didn't get through.

I am certain that there is a policy somewhere that says that this must happen, but it was so rare, it was almost laughable. I did laugh when Stuart in rehab used to come in, pick up my wrist and say "You are still Keith". It's a discipline that is well worth following! Additionally, Stuart was meticulous about spelling out the name of and dosage of each medication, and what it was for. We never had a problem with him, but later in our experience, not in rehab, a nurse came in and started laying out all the medications and said "Your doctor switched you to Heparin instead of Lovonox." Claire asked her "Why?" and she looked at her like she had spoken Greek, and answered "I don't know." Claire said "I don't want him to have it until I know why he is getting it." The nurse said "OK, but I will have to call him" and left. About 15 minutes later she came back in and said casually "I have the Lovonox. The Heparin was for another patient." I only hope and pray that this is not a normal occurrence and it troubles me enormously that were we not intelligent, observant and resourceful this kind of thing might have been very serious. That was not the last time that something like this happened.

After the three ghosts had come and gone, it was time for my breakfast. Food was delivered on a tray, and since I was on steroids, I had a rapacious appetite. I was like Cookie Monster in an Oreo Factory. I wanted to eat everything, even the tasteless stuff they put on my tray.

I was hungry, and I was on an unrestricted diet. I craved cheese, but that wasn't on the menu, and for a breakfast appetizer I could chose orange slices, orange juice, prunes or jook. I didn't have any idea what jook was apart from a 15 point word score in Scrabble but I found out later that jook was an Asian dish that includes rice, some meat, and sounded totally unappetizing to me, but I guess ravioli sounds yucky to them).

I saw some food like it when I was in China, when I discovered the meaning of the word "execrable". We were going on a Yangtze River Cruise as a part of our adventure in China, and happened to look in a tour book to see what we could expect. The tour book stated that the food on the Yangtze cruise was "execrable" and as neither Claire nor I knew what this word meant, we looked around the book store for a dictionary, and finding one, discovered that "execrable" means "inedible." It really gave us something to look forward to, and was a joke for the next three days! Jook sounded just like it. I grew up in England, the Royal Center of Bland Cuisine, and this sounded even blander!

I could have all the prunes I wanted! In my brain I knew how good prunes were for your digestive system, but the only things I didn't like about prunes were the way they looked, the way they smelled and the way they tasted. I suppose if I was really desperate, the way you might be after three weeks of survival training in the sub arctic tundra, or like I was when nothing was moving through my digestive system, then prunes would be the breakfast of champions, but as long as that day didn't come I would be avoiding them, and since they didn't do any good that I could see during my recent need, that just reinforced my "anti-prune" stand.

What was the point of my having great blood test results, with low triglycerides, and low cholesterol, if I couldn't eat good food. Now, I was paralyzed in the hospital, losing weight like crazy, pumped up on steroids, and my ravenous appetite was not being satisfied. My body was crying out for food. Not only did my breakfast not come up to my basic minimum standards, but it also came up late. Typically it was served between 8:30 and 9, and that was over three hours after my morning alarm, the dawn chorus of massed staplers.

I was often roused from night of sleep by the sound of multiple stacks of papers being stapled together by a stapler that didn't have sufficient capacity for the papers it was being asked to hold together. This was the sheaves of papers with all the medications ordered, the tests ordered, and the other orders on each patient that the nurses had to carry around with them since they didn't have WOWs, so this was my morning alarm clock.

My solution to the problem of late breakfast was to ask for snack bars that I could eat when I woke up to stave off the pangs of hunger before breakfast arrived. Then I could wait for the tray. The process for ordering food was interesting. When the breakfast tray arrived, there was a blank menu for the next day on it. No pencil, just a menu. Sometimes, if I wasn't sufficiently careful, it was a wet and pulpy menu. I could circle things on the menu and the following day they would arrive.

For breakfast I could choose from three kinds of cereals including oatmeal, and I generally selected Raisin Bran, but it took me a couple of days to figure out that if I did, I also had to specify that I needed milk. Apparently the kitchen staff assumed nothing.

If you didn't circle it on the menu you didn't get it. If it wasn't there to circle, you had to write it in. Yes, I was told you could write stuff in on the menu, and this was true, but it didn't matter, because the kitchen would only deliver the things that were circled. No one told me that you had to write things in and then circle them! I found this out when they gave me a copy of what I ordered and the banana that I had been looking forward to eating with my Raisin Bran and fat free milk was missing in action despite being written on the menu.

I began to figure the system out when I got my hamburger with no condiments. It was a bun and a burger. Claire was able to go down to the cafeteria and get me lettuce, tomato, ketchup, mustard, mayonnaise and relish, and while she was down there she asked a man behind the counter about the practice. The cook told her that the policy was to never second guess the patient, so we learned that if we wanted something we had to write it in and circle it. The next day I wrote in my banana, drew a picture of what it should look like, and circled it clearly. I was going to color it yellow so that there could be no misunderstanding, but they had no colored crayons at the nurses' station, so I had no idea how they kept children amused while they were waiting for food to be delivered. Also, just because you ordered it and circled it, that didn't mean that you would always get it. Several times decaf tea arrived without the tea bag (maybe that was their idea of decaf tea), and I couldn't tell the difference between their decaf coffee and a mug of hot water.

The cereal course was followed by pancakes (just average) or French toast, which was actually pretty good, and something called hot syrup, which I believe was composed entirely of chemicals and could not even remember meeting a maple tree in springtime. I could also have a bagel and cream cheese, but eventually we figured out that if I ordered that, Claire could eat it, and save us a fortune on her breakfast. Eggs were an option, but despite the battery operated hot plate, they generally arrived lukewarm, and bacon was almost never an option.

The food always sounded better than it tasted; they had obviously hired a professional menu writer who knew that it was always good to describe a bunch of lettuce leaves and one miniature tomato as a tossed green salad. The menu writer didn't understand the basic principle of customer service: Underpromise and over deliver. This creates reasonable expectations on the part of the customer, and then the customer is pleasantly surprised when these expectations are exceeded. Of course now I began to see a big flaw in the system. If I was in a different hospital yesterday, then I didn't get a menu for today, so I couldn't choose what I wanted, and instead I was given whatever no one else had ordered or the stuff that the lady/man in this bed before me selected before he/she transferred or whatever.

I did however discover that there was a snack cart that made the rounds twice a day! This never happened in the ICU! I quickly made friends with Kip, the snack cart guy! He was charming, personable, and I couldn't imagine anyone not being happy to see him, but Claire, in her own personable style, asked him once if people were ever nasty to him, and he said that they were! She couldn't believe it, but he said that if a patient was having a bad day they might take it out on anyone, and he was no exception! I never did anything to upset Kip! Once I discovered that I could get something from the snack cart whenever he came around, he was my main man! One of the nurses even wrote a sign for my door, "Always offer snacks, even when his door is closed and he appears to be asleep". I never minded being awoken by Kip!

He would also offer snacks to Claire! Kip quickly learned of Claire's preference for chocolate chip cookies, and always had one for her if there was one in the kitchen, and when we saw his smiling face twice a day as he came by with the cart, it was like a ray of sunshine. He probably did more for our spirits than anyone! It was a joy, twice a day!

My other saving grace was Claire, who was allowed on the outside, to go to real shops and buy real food, like chocolate and cheese and crackers, and occasional goodies like pizza, hamburgers, fries, milk shakes, crepes and cinnamon rolls, and bring them in to me, which she did, regularly!

During the afternoon of Day 16 my second plasmapheresis treatment took place, this time with a different technician, Marcella. She was full of information about how the process worked; she had many years of experience as a registered nurse and had become fascinated by the plasmapheresis treatments, and had at one time been involved in the marketing of the equipment, so she knew how to deal with people and she knew her subject, two great assets for anyone who wants to succeed at business. She informed us that there was another patient in the hospital with TM, and she acknowledged just how unusual this was! TM is very rare, so what were the chances of there being two patients with TM in the same hospital at the same time? We asked her to please ask the other patient if she would be interested in a "peer visit", and she said she would, even though we knew that this was probably against every hospital policy that ever existed, but if we could do it, we wanted to!

We were very encouraged by the results we were seeing from the plasmapheresis, but we were learning way more about how hospitals work than we had any interest in knowing. Our primary areas of expertise prior to this had been teaching workshops on customer service in retail and manufacturing, not in hospital care, yet the principles were the same, and the process issues abounded, so it was nearly impossible for us not to see some things that could be done better!

For example, I know that when a new patient is admitted to a unit, they must first be settled in their room, be introduced to their nursing team, and have their medical needs taken care of, but it would be great if they could be shown or told the process for ordering their food, and invited to do so. It is so much more respectful than to just bring a tray of assorted food without considering their preferences.

It was also great when we figured out that we could ask the doctor for a "do not disturb" order. My vital signs were stable and many of my functions were being tracked automatically by a remote monitoring device, so I was able to get more rest when I asked to be disturbed as little as possible and the doctor actually made it an order.

Chapter 6 – The Roller Coaster Ride

Day 17

Today I stood up, for the first time, by the side of my bed, with a physical therapist on one side and an occupational therapist on the other. I actually stood for about three minutes, and my blood pressure stayed in the normal range. I was overjoyed, delighted, elated, and encouraged by this achievement because it meant that I still had some muscles in my legs, and that the potential existed for me to walk again! I was definitely shaky, but it sure felt good to be vertical after 16 days of lying on my back. I also still had my sense of "proprioception"; this is the ability of the brain to detect where limbs are located in space, and it is necessary to walk effectively. I could feel my feet beneath me, I knew where they were, and they were supporting me! My muscles were weak, they had basically disappeared, but there was promise that they could come back!

As usual, the Dream Team came to visit, and were astounded by how much stronger I was. It was easy to attribute it to the plasmapheresis, but I am certain that the combination of steroids, physical therapy as well as my own exercises were in part responsible. We had a lot to celebrate, and Claire enabled my celebration by providing me with chocolate, something else that was conspicuous by its absence from the hospital food menus. Haven't they heard about the amazing antioxidants that are contained in dark chocolate, and how chocolate can help sick people get well? As far as I am concerned, chocolate should be one of the four basic elements on the food pyramid, together with potato chips, ice cream, and strawberries. I would even consider it a complete meal if you could combine those four basic ingredients in any combination and add decaffeinated coffee (preferably tasty). Being in the hospital gives you time to reflect on all these important issues. I knew about Maslow and his hierarchy of human needs. I had gone right back to the essential primitive basic survival and physiological needs, of food, water, shelter, security, coffee and internet access. Never mind self actualization! I hoped that one day soon I would be moving up the pyramid and getting back to the life that I considered normal.

I asked myself what had happened to me on July 20th. It felt to me as though I had been attacked. I decided that "attack" was the right word to use to describe what had happened to me on July 20th, after all it seemed to fit the circumstances far better than the other words that came to mind, words like "event", "onset", "incident", "episode", "beginning" etc. This was definitely a "way of life" changing event, and things would never be quite the same again. I had been attacked, without warning, without any apparent provocation, and my life would be changed, perhaps permanently. I was really hoping and praying that after the rehab process was complete I would have most of my normal bodily functions restored yet I knew inherently that there might always be some residual concerns to deal with.

In my research I had discovered that TM is "normally" a one-time event, and that once you had dealt with it, it was not likely to reoccur. I say likely, because sometimes it is the first attack of multiple sclerosis, which is a permanent disorder of the spinal cord, and we learned later there are cases of recurring TM and also of relapsing TM, not that I had been given a choice, but I was nevertheless relieved that I had what appeared to be the single episode version. I knew, thanks to the success I had already had, that I had the possibility of complete rehabilitation.

TM is a disorder not a disease. Both disorders and diseases can be treated, but "disease" sounds like something that might be contagious, so I had to assure my family and in particular my grandchildren, that what I had could not be spread by contact, that it did not run in our family, it was highly unlikely that they would get it, and more importantly that their Nana (Claire) wouldn't get it. I was just the "lucky" one who got it. Unlike Job's friends who asked him what he had done to piss God off so much, I was not about to ask this question. My life was full of things which I am sure hadn't pleased God, but I had long ago asked for his mercy and forgiveness, and knew that He had given me his Grace. Now I had this gift and it was up to me to make a blessing of it. Anyone can steer a ship in calm waters, but the true test of seamanship comes when the waters get rough and dangerous. This was a test, and I intended to excel!

Day 18

After my normal daily routine of visits from the friendly vampire, the Dream Team and the nurse of the day, I was informed that my plasmapheresis would have to be delayed because my lab results showed that my fibrinogen levels were too low. Evidently this was one of the reasons for the blood suckers every day, although I didn't know this, and truth be known, I didn't even know what fibrinogen was; I had absolutely no clue what they were talking about! Once again, Google came to our rescue and we learned that fibrinogen is a clotting agent in the blood, and whether or not you can take the plasma away during plasmapheresis depends on the blood's ability to clot. I was informed that the lab would do a retest, and depending on the results I may or may not be able to have the treatment. While we waited for the results of the second test, I sat there in bed willing my fibrinogens to go forth and multiply.

In the meantime we continued to exercise, enjoy our access to the internet, play games on our Nintendo DS's, and generally keep ourselves upbeat. Later in the day we got the results from the second test, and it showed that the first blood test was

WRONG! My fibrinogen levels were actually fine, but now it was too late to proceed with the plasmapheresis; the schedule was already changed, and this was very disappointing because it meant that it delayed my transfer back to rehab by yet another day.

I realized once again that I was not in control. It didn't matter what test results showed, God was in control. We had been away from home, from friends, from family for two and a half weeks now, when we had planned to be away only 3 days. We had received several care packages, some lovely fruit, cheese and crackers, shortbread cookies, tea, biscotti, truffles, and other goodies, as well as flowers but there was nothing that anyone could send me that would placate my growing need to be well enough to be out of the hospital and back to rehab, because I was certain that it was only through the professional care of the therapists there that I would truly be "made well" and be strong enough to go home!

Day 19

There is a different atmosphere in a hospital on weekends; the regular crew we saw during the week was home spending their weekend with their families, and although there are some who enjoy working weekends and nights, we found that often hospitals would use "floaters" in from other units and agency nurses, on weekends. It must be a nightmare to keep a hospital running; it is so dependent on people in every possible line of work, and scheduling people for weekends must be even more difficult.

For the patient, there were fewer visits from travelling groups of doctors on the weekends, and there was hardly any physical or occupational therapy, so we were pretty much left to our own devices. In my case, I was feeling so good, and NOT getting any real therapy, that it left me feeling once again that my time was being wasted. I had been told by my therapists in rehab that I should NOT be doing any exercises between my sessions with them; that it was important to get my rest in between therapies, but there I was getting four sessions a day. Here, in the hospital, there was so little therapy, and I felt great (other than my inability to walk, or feel pain or temperature below the rib cage) so I wanted everything to be more normal, or at least be geared to getting me out of here and back to rehab.

Claire and I took some time to catch up on some things that we hadn't had time for before. She cut my hair and trimmed my beard, and gave me a bed bath (which I think would have felt good if I could have felt it!) I wasn't allowed to shower because of the vascular catheter, and so this was the best I could do. As she washed my legs she asked me if the cloth was hot or cold and I had absolutely no idea. Everything felt the same temperature. My temperature nerves were sending spurious signals, my buttocks felt like I had wicked sunburn, my legs felt cold to the touch and my feet were burning up. This had all started on July 20th and hadn't changed since! It was not painful, just mildly irritating like pins and needles. I was pleased, however, when I could tell the difference on my leg between a face cloth and a towel. I had retained my "soft touch" sensation, and I knew this could be useful, but at the moment I was stumped in terms of when and how.

We talked about the changes we had planned to make in the house. I was doing so well with my recovery that we decided to hold off the people who were itching to build a wheelchair ramp for our house. We were pleased that our friends had gone in and reinforced the railings on the staircases, and they had also moved a bed into our living room, so we felt that the house was good enough for us to go back to, and knew that we would figure out the rest when we got home.

111

In the afternoon, during my third plasmapheresis treatment, my immunologist Dr. Hawkins came in. I had plenty of questions for him: I wanted to know what the "ideal" number of plasmapheresis treatments was and what would happen to my immune system once I finished the treatments and the steroids. I was so intent on talking to him, that the alarms kept going off on the plasmapheresis machine. My vocal chords were so close to my jugular vein, that even when I wasn't talking, but just saying "Uh hum" the vein would constrict, and the fluid would stop flowing, so Claire finally stepped in and told me to stop talking, but she continued to talk, and I got to listen, and all our questions were answered.

It was one of the things that I really valued about the doctors I had in this hospital. They might not know the answers to the questions I had (in particular, every intern left with a list of questions to research) but if they did know the answer, they left no iota of information out. We got full information from every single doctor.

Day 20

Clearly something was working. Each morning I woke feeling stronger than the day before, and this morning I was ready for anything! We had another full day plus some before I would have another treatment, and we were looking for something to do, so when we received a phone call from the plasmapheresis technician, Marcella, who had told us that there was another TM patient in the hospital, we were anxious to hear what the verdict was regarding a "peer visit"! Marcella told us that she had spoken with Rosie, the other TM patient, and she was eager to meet with us. Now we had to explore hospital policies regarding cross ward visitation, but apparently if both patients agreed, and there was no medical reason why a patient couldn't go off the unit, then there was no problem. We asked for, and received permission to disconnect the remote telemetry unit that enabled the nurses to monitor my vital signs, and Claire helped me transfer into the wheelchair. We were on our way to another ward, another floor, another environment, and another source of information about this disorder.

We had been given Rosie's room number, so we took the elevator to the right level and Claire wheeled me to the room. Rosie was in the middle of a plasmapheresis treatment with Marcella, and was reading a magazine. Her room was even smaller than mine was, and her husband was there with her, so there wasn't enough room in there for all of us, so Claire wheeled me in, and then she invited Rosie's husband, to come out into the hallway to chat. After our visit, when we had discussed what we had learned, it was very similar! Claire had focused more on the impact on family and friends, and I had focused on Rosie's symptoms and treatment, and when we compared notes, the story looked like this:

Rosie, was about my age, and had been struck by TM in September of the previous year but had not been correctly diagnosed until two months later. Her paralysis wasn't as severe as mine, and her lesions were not on the same vertebrae as mine were, so she was far more physically capable than I was, but despite that, she had been in and out of the hospital ever since. She had been on steroids, but they never made her fully well, so now she was on plasmapheresis for the first time, and she was considering becoming part of a clinical trial to test whether a drug that was used to treat non-Hodgkin's lymphoma would actually be beneficial to patients with MS and TM. I was interested in this study because the drug was manufactured by one of the companies that I did work for. Rosie could actually walk, and often did up and down the hospital corridors, usually holding on to the rails in the hallway, and she could do a lot of her normal household chores at home as well, but she was anxious to get as much healing as possible. She had received outpatient physical therapy, and was satisfied with her progress. She was now in the hospital for the same reason I was, for plasmapheresis.

Rosie's husband was retired and quite knowledgeable about the disorder by this time; of course they had lived with it for nearly a year already, and among other things, he had retired from the local transportation authority, so he offered to get Claire a map of the transit system to make her ability to travel around easier! She was thrilled! My resourceful wife had gotten herself a monthly bus pass, which allowed her infinite rides on any of the San Francisco busses. She was already quite the expert, but with a map she would be invincible. At about supper time we went back to the unit, and the nurse hooked me back up to all of my monitors, and we talked about all we had learned, and once again were amazed to learn how uniquely this disorder behaves in each individual.

Day 21

Today started out as a bonanza day, with a visit from Dr. Tabitha of the Dream Team who brought us another piece of important information. She told me that the New England Journal of Medicine had just published an article about TM, and that she had downloaded a copy of the article for me to read. It was very interesting; it was written to help primary care physicians diagnose TM so that effective treatment could begin as soon as the disorder was confirmed. Based on my ER experience I knew that most doctors wouldn't connect the dots, so I was really pleased that such a pre-eminent journal had given it attention.

During physical therapy, with Susan on one side and another therapist on the other, I had a chance to stand and to take my

first steps with a walker, and actually managed to wa⌐
the nurses' station once, sitting every few steps to re-⌐
in the wheelchair that Claire pushed behind me. It was
to be vertical and I was very excited. If I could walk with
walker, well, that was nearly normal! It was also clear from the
faces of the nursing staff and from the response of Susan, that
everyone was thrilled with my progress. At the end of the day,
however, things went seriously downhill.

My plasmapheresis treatment was scheduled for 5:00 pm but it
didn't start until 7:00 pm, as the technician (Franklin, the same
technician who had done the first treatment in the ICU) was
missing one of the materials that he needed to complete the
process. So it was after dinner when the material arrived and
Franklin started. Almost immediately I began to feel hot and
clammy, and beads of sweat were running down my neck. I
asked Franklin to ring for my nurse, and Grace, one of my
favorites, arrived. I told her that I was concerned and asked her
for a cold damp face cloth, which she quickly provided for me. I
wiped the sweat away, but it didn't seem to help, so I told
Franklin that I really didn't feel well. After a further 10 minutes
I began to feel a tightening in my chest, and felt the need to
cough. Something was impacting my lungs, and I felt short of
breath, as though I could not get a full breath. I told Franklin
once again that I didn't feel well, and demanded a nurse right
away. He ignored me, and just kept watching over the machine,
carrying on with the procedure. Once again, I repeated my
request for a nurse and demanded that a doctor be called NOW,
raising my voice for added urgency, and this time he actually did
respond, going out of the room and asking for Grace. When he
returned, I asked him if there was any risk associated with
terminating the process, and he told me that there wasn't, so
when Grace came in, and I told her what had been happening,
she agreed that the process should stop immediately, and she

ordered 2 liters of oxygen to be delivered, which helped to ease my respiratory distress.

Franklin disconnected the tubes from my neck and sealed up the vascular catheter, but of course the tubes were full of blood which hadn't yet been recycled into me, so as he removed them, my blood went everywhere! It was not pleasant for anyone at that point, but once the process stopped I began to feel a little more normal, and could have a conversation with Grace about what had happened. She had her own observations, and reported that I was "diaphoretic, tachycardic, and dyspneic" which meant I was sweating profusely, had an accelerated heart rate, and was having difficulty breathing. She called for the doctor and within 10 minutes the doctor on duty came and ordered an EKG, which fortunately showed that my heart was beating normally and the oxygen level in my blood stream was normal.

By 7:45 pm my vital signs were all stable and my body had returned to normal. Franklin was still there, so I asked him to tell me what was different about this treatment from my previous three treatments, and he replied "nothing, everything was the same as before". Having had asthma as an allergic reaction to the inert ingredient in my generic anti-seizure medication as well as having been allergic to animals and other substances since I was a child, I suspected that I had an allergic reaction to something used during plasmapheresis, and I thought that it might have been something in the Albumin that was being used, so I asked Grace to hold the partially used bottle and do a lot trace on the unit. Grace took the bottle and sent it to the lab for analysis, and also asked the pharmacy if there was a difference in batch or lot number from those used during my previous treatments. The pharmacy informed her that the batch of Albumin used in my treatment was from the same manufacturing batch as those used in all previous treatments; that in fact, they had been using the same batch all week with no problems.

I am sure that Franklin was certified to use the plasmapheresis machine. I am sure that he had proven that he had the technical expertise to connect the bottles and lines, to turn the dials, and to run a normal plasmapheresis process, but he wasn't prepared to handle my adverse reaction. It appeared that he neither expected, nor was trained to respond to this condition that might occur once in 5000 times, and that was frightening. If I hadn't taken such assertive action, the process may have ended very badly.

When I got to speak with Dr. Hawkins, my immunologist, the following day I discovered that there were some rare instances when patients had an allergic reaction during plasmapheresis, and that as a precaution the patient could be pre-medicated with intravenous Benadryl. He also advised me that in the unlikely event that I needed further plasmapheresis treatments I should insist on the pre-medication and that under no circumstances should I use Albumin products from the same company that I had this reaction to. When everything had stabilized and the technician had left, I called Claire at her hotel to let her know what had happened. She was terribly concerned, and advised me to write everything down right away while I remembered it, and to save it for future reference, so I did, and I asked her to please come in early the next morning, so that she would be here when we were discussing the next steps with the doctors.

Day 22

Claire arrived early as she had promised, and as the doctors came in, one by one, we had to repeat what had happened the previous night to each new doctor. They offered five possible causes of the reaction: A simple calcium deficiency (plasmapheresis depletes the amount of calcium in the blood); an allergic reaction to the Albumin; an allergic reaction to the blood thinning agent used during the process; a shock reaction to the amount of blood being taken out during the process (possibly dehydration), or a pulmonary embolism.

No one knew for certain what the cause was, but ultimately, after a full consultation between the immunologist, the hospitalist, and the neurologist, we all agreed that it was most likely an allergic reaction to the Albumin. Apparently this occurs in about 1 in 5000 plasmapheresis treatments. We also found out that what I had experienced was a stage two allergic response. Normally stage 1 would be an itchiness of the skin which would then be followed, if nothing changed, by a stage 2 reaction which could include a respiratory problem. In my case I had gone straight to stage 2, or perhaps I simply hadn't noticed any itchiness since I still had no sensation from the chest down. Now it was up to my immunologist and my neurologist to decide the next step.

They spent a good deal of time talking before they decided to discontinue the plasmapheresis and transfer me back to the rehab center for further therapy. I was really glad to have the decision made, and know that now we could get on with recovery, which had seemed to be going so well in the rehab center. Despite all the chaos, I still had my physical therapy, during which I actually stood and took a few steps without the aid of the walker, and I got a bonus session in the afternoon, during which I walked around the nurses' station with a walker, more secure in my steps and much stronger! After all this exercise, though, I was exhausted and ready for bed.

Day 23

It was Wednesday, the decision had been made to terminate the plasmapheresis, and I was ready to be transferred back to the rehab center. The discharge order was put in, the doctors all came by to say goodbye, and I had my last session of physical therapy during which I impressed the whole medical staff by my ability to walk down the hall twice, with no walker, holding on to the railing, and even crossing open doorways unassisted where there was no railing. As is our practice, when we are travelling or relocating we get prepared early, and make sure that everything is ready in plenty of time, but as the day wore on it became increasingly obvious that the transfer would not be happening quickly, so I reluctantly prepared to spend yet another night in the hospital waiting for the powers that be to make and execute a simple decision.

Suddenly and totally unexpectedly, my urethra suddenly opened! Remember, I had been intermittently catheterized for the last 23 days, so it was a shock to find myself actually urinating! This was apparently a result of the medication "Flowmax" that I had been given, actually, since the beginning of this adventure. It was suddenly working! For twelve straight hours I was peeing like a racehorse, with no end in sight. I spent all night clutching a urinal between my legs, and in the morning I noticed that I had rubbed the skin of my inner thighs totally raw. It was yet another example of how because my skin couldn't detect pain I could easily and unwittingly hurt myself. Claire, appalled, set off on a mission to find me a better urinal.

When she found one she discovered that at least as far as the cost to her, a consumer, the cost for a urinal exactly like the one I had in the hospital, and the cost of one with a smooth rim, were identical!

Regardless, it was great to finally be urinating on my own and possibly get off catheterization, but true to form, and never one to be satisfied with just SOME improvement, I wanted it ALL. I wanted to actually control the flow. I was thinking of asking the doctor for a lower dosage of Flowmax, or if perhaps there was a medicine called "flow medium" or even a double dose of "flow light", but no such products existed.

I was still contemplating the vagaries of modern medicine when Dr. Graham came in. I handed him the New England Journal of Medicine article that Dr. Tabitha had given to me; he took the article and read it thoroughly before handing it back to me, declaring that the article was not written for neurologists. I was really glad that he knew far more than the article, it meant my nerves were in good hands!

Day 24

I had now had a discharge order from the hospital back to rehab for a full day, and yet.....I was still in the hospital! The nurses had decided to put me on a condom catheter, which enabled me to stop constantly using the urinal, although Claire had found a urinal without the rough plastic flashing on the outside of the rim and had also cut one of my rubber bottom socks and slid the top of the sock over the opening of the urinal to add yet another layer of protection. It was that rough edge on the outside of the rim opening that had ripped my skin to shreds, Needless to say, she used a sharpie to write ALL OVER the urinal, that it was my personal property!

The same doctors who said goodbye to me the previous day, came by again, and asked me why I was still there. I explained that I was still waiting for GIC to approve my transfer back to the rehab center. It was now Thursday, the weekend was coming, and Claire and I were getting very frustrated because we had heard nothing, and there was no update from anyone. It was as frustrating as sitting on a plane and being told by the captain that takeoff has been delayed, but giving no reason for the delay and no estimate for when takeoff might actually occur.

While we were seething in frustration, a woman came in from the health and healing group. This group offered complimentary services to patients, and I had already had a massage from them and now I was being offered an opportunity to use some art to help my healing. When the woman asked me how I was feeling, I answered "my legs don't feel at all, but my brain is mad as hell, and my hands want to throttle someone!" She suggested that perhaps drawing a picture could help express my feelings.

I explained that I had been waiting more than 24 hours to get approval from my insurance company for a transfer back to the rehab center where I might ACTUALLY get BETTER, but that it hadn't happened yet. Then I had a great idea, and I asked if she had any clay or any other material I could use to make a voodoo doll that I could then stick pins in. "That might help me" I said! She allowed that unfortunately, she didn't have any materials with her other than paper and drawing supplies, but that I was welcome to draw a picture if I thought that might help! I thought about drawing a picture of an insurance representative hanging on a scaffold, but realized that this was not a very Christian thing to wish for. Oddly, she left fairly quickly after that.

Claire was tired of it, so she decided to call the insurance company case manager directly to find out what the problem was. After an hour she got a call back. It turned out that our case manager had been on bereavement leave, and had just returned that morning. We felt badly for her, and Claire expressed the appropriate sentiments, but apparently, although this was not confirmed with her, there was no one in the office who knew about our case or could handle our case in her absence. Now she was back and getting up to speed on the issues. She probably overstepped her authority, but she verbally approved the transfer, and a transfer was scheduled for 4:00 pm. Sure enough, the ambulance and EMTs showed up on time, and the nurses removed the IV line, the doctor re-signed the discharge papers, and once again we were headed to rehab.

Every disappointing experience we had, other than those directly related to my health over which we had minimal control, usually boiled down to some kind of process or policy issue. It was nearly always about some policy that didn't always make sense, some technique that didn't always work, some training that wasn't sufficient, some management style that wasn't effective, or some other decision made that didn't focus on the right outcome. In a hospital there should be only one outcome driving every single process, decision, management action, technique, and training: the health of the patient. If something is being done that isn't motivated by that desired outcome then it had better be totally neutral to the health of the patient, and, every patient is unique!

I was certainly unique (in fact, I hate being called "normal"). My disorder was rare, my strength was excellent, my spirits were high, my motivation to get well was through the roof, my intellect was superb, and thanks to the internet my access to information was nearly unsurpassed. "Normal" processes didn't exactly fit my idea of how things should work. Add to all of that the fact that we get paid for telling people how to do things more efficiently and more effectively. The hospital and the insurance company had their hands full with us, and we had our hands full with them!

I know that not every patient will have the resources to comprehend all the varied aspects of his/her disease, disorder, illness, injury, or treatment, and therefore it takes a lot of savvy for a physician to balance the value of his/her time against the ability of the patient to understand all the information the doctor has. In our case, there was never a moment when the doctors didn't take all the time required to fully answer our questions. I can only assume that we had shown ourselves able to both assimilate it and make good use of it in our own work to get me well, but we never felt that we were kept from any important information regarding my health, and I even sometimes felt that in my overwhelming thirst for information I was keeping the doctors talking with us far longer than was really necessary, but they never ever made us feel as though they didn't have all the time in the world for us! For that, we were intensely grateful!

Chapter 7 - Back to Rehab

Day 24 - Continued

I was very pleased to see the hospital, from my vantage point in the back of the ambulance, as it faded away in the distance behind us. This was a definitely a trip in the right direction. I knew that I would experience the very best recovery in the rehab center with people who were totally focused on getting me independent.

When I arrived back at the rehab center I discovered that I had been upgraded to a larger room with the best view in the facility! It was a terrific room! We were totally happy. Claire had managed to get the suitcases transported in the ambulance with me, and she unpacked my things and put everything away. We were much closer to her hotel, so instead of a 90 minute bus trip on two busses each way, she would take one train two stops to the front door of her hotel. Things were definitely looking up!

Except - - there was no internet access in the room!

Surprise, surprise! Remember, they had to switch the Ethernet port on in the room before, so we had to get them to do the same in this room as well! This time, Claire knew the phone number of the clinic manager, and called him directly. We had internet within 30 minutes, although we didn't get told that it was switched on; Claire just kept trying to get access, and suddenly it worked!

Once again, Aaron the admissions nurse checked us in, and Claire filled in the inventory report. This time we had a lot less "stuff" and it all fit on one page! Claire never told Aaron that he had never picked up the last report, and we suspected that he wouldn't get this one either. We just laughed about it. It felt really good to be back in familiar territory once more. Our nurse, Judy, was cheerful and chatty, and as we got to know more about her, it turned out that she was married to the first nurse I had in the TICU in the hospital we had just come from! It made a nice connection for us!

Day 25

The next day my schedule was posted on my wall on time, and showed two sessions of occupational therapy, two sessions of physical therapy, plus one session with the psychiatrist, and one with the speech therapist. It was going to be a busy day! It almost seemed like "normal".

Our room had one chair, almost a lounger, so it was not the right kind of chair for me to sit in and actually do anything, but normal wasn't lying around in bed between activities, so we got an upright chair from the activity room, or went to the activity room and I spent less time in bed, and more time sitting upright. That was more normal as well.

I got up and dressed myself before it was time for my first session of occupational therapy, and when Miriam came in she was thrilled to see that I was clearly doing well. I had started dressing in my own clothes as soon as I could. This made things more normal as well, plus I didn't look like a patient; I was wearing a t-shirt and shorts and I looked like I was on holiday instead of seriously ill. Everything that could be done to approximate normal was done! After my shower (initially I was "authorized" a shower three times a week, and generally in the evenings since the staff's activity level was greater in the mornings, but I had been cleared to shower by myself, so that was terrific!) Miriam outfitted me with the equipment that I needed to get around in rehab, and funnily, this time, they

didn't issue me an electric wheelchair! I think I had terr
them sufficiently the last time so they decided to "grounc
(so to speak). It was time for me to learn how to use a mar.
wheelchair, as well as a walker and a cane. I soon got used to
the wheelchair and I was really glad that I had invested some
energy in strengthening my upper body, because even with the
weight I had lost, I was still a heavy load to push around!

For physical therapy I used my walker to walk down to the gym.
Karen, also really pleased that I hadn't regressed during my time
away) gave me an assessment test. This was the test the
insurance companies used to determine when it was time to go
home. I was really pleased, as I scored 37 points out of a
possible 56. Things I was able to do: I stood up for one minute
unsupported with my eyes shut; I bent down and picked up a
box of tissues from the floor, also unsupported and I walked up
and down a small flight of stairs with the aid of a cane. Then
Karen put a small step stool in front of me, and asked me if I
could step on to it and step back down off of it without support.

I looked at the step and it might as well have been Mount
Everest for all the chance I had of doing what she asked, but we
both celebrated that I had not only not lost ground during my
hospital stay, but actually came back even stronger than I had
been before I left. When I left, I couldn't even walk! After
therapy, and all the exercising I had done, I still had the strength
and energy to walk back to my room with only the aid of my
walker.

My next visitors were another neuropsychologist (she decided
that my brain was still OK in spite of what many people might
have thought), the speech therapist (who was again
disappointed to discover that her services were not required),
and most surprisingly the clinic manager, who actually came by
to thank us for kicking up such a stink about the lack of internet

access. He told us that technicians were coming in the very next week to install wireless routers throughout the floor so that every room would have high speed wireless access. He also told us that this had been a project that had been waiting for over a year, ever since the huge rehab, and had simply never been done. This was in part, of course, because Claire got so "intensely" involved and made it her issue, but it also turned out that another patient came in shortly after me, and railed at the lack of internet access, so the two-front approach certainly made things happen.

I made full use of my new found ability and connected with my grandchildren online, and we had dinner together, in spite of the time and distance between us. It was fun to pretend we were having a meal together, as we ate our own food in separate places linked by the wonders of webcams.

Before I went to sleep for the night one of my favorite nurses (and, as I have said, there were many "favorites") Irma came in with a special treat – Trader Joe's Bittersweet Chocolate with Almonds, and she gave me a big piece. This chocolate comes from Belgium and was (and still is) absolutely outstanding, so we started a conversation about chocolate that went on quite a while, since we were both big fans!

Day 26

I hadn't had any pain in days, so it was about time for two sessions with Greg, who told me that if he focused on the areas of muscle weakness, then I would get more movement back. In the absence of an alternative I decided to agree with him, but I complained about his harsh methods during my daily Facebook updates, and I had a number of people comment back that they could use someone like Greg as their personal trainer, someone to "kick their butts". After two sessions with Greg I could hardly move, so I came back to my room, and enjoyed my first nap with my wife since this whole ordeal had begun. She just closed the door, and climbed up into the bed with me, and it felt so very good to hold her in my arms again after 25 days and nights of separation.

After our nap I was on the internet once again, and this time I discovered that a book had been written about one person's experience with transverse myelitis. The book was called "Scrambled Leggs" by Sally Franz. Claire opened her Kindle, turned on the wireless network, found the book, downloaded it, and began reading it aloud to me within two and a half minutes from the time I mentioned it. Now that is technology!

I was fascinated by the parallels between Sally's experience and mine. She had been skiing down a mountain when her leg became numb and turned to mush beneath her, and I knew that feeling. Sally also described the sensation in her legs as though she "had a wicked sunburn or was being stung by a 1000 bees", and I knew that feeling as well. It was great to connect that way with someone who had documented their experience so that it could be shared with others, and that was when Claire and I had the first glimmer of an idea about writing this book. We had been keeping a diary since nearly the beginning of this adventure, and we knew that we had some great stories to share.

My temperature receptors had been rewired; my hot water sensor was in the cold water pipe and the cold water sensor was in the hot water one, and it didn't make any sense to me. My feet felt like they were on fire all the time, my legs felt cold and as though my skin was not really mine. I could touch my skin, and feel the pressure of the touch, but it felt as though the sense was dulled, almost as though my nerves were suddenly hidden deeply below the surface somewhere. I wanted to test it, so I put an ice cube on my leg and watched as it melted, but it never felt at all cold on my skin. I could feel the weight of the ice cube and sense the water dripping off of my leg, but it certainly did not feel like it should have. I wondered what use this new condition might be, and realized that one benefit would be that I could go swimming in the ocean in York Beach, Maine without getting frostbite! Most people don't even put their feet in the water without wet suits, and really brave people go into the ocean almost all the way up to their knees in the summertime (but they are usually Canadian).

Day 27

I woke up early and took advantage of the time zone difference to Skype with my mother in England and also with my daughter and her family before their breakfast. My grandson was pleased, because now he could see me, and he could show me the things he was playing with. He told me that he was teaching his Dad how Bob the Builder could become Dennis the Destroyer! That's a four year old for you! At about 9:00 am, my nurse came in and gave me my morning meds, which included my daily shot of Lovonox. The shot was always given in my stomach, and for the first time since the attack I felt the sharp needle being inserted on my left side approximately at the navel level. It might have been the first time a patient was thrilled with a painful shot! It meant that some sensation was coming back!

Since it was Sunday, I had only one scheduled activity and that was occupational therapy with Miriam. We walked into the unit kitchen to see how I could manage there, and I did everything she asked me to. She asked me to get things out of the refrigerator and then she told me to put them back, and when I asked her why she kept changing her mind, she told me that it was all a part of occupational therapy; she was trying to get me used to living in a house with someone who might be indecisive (she obviously didn't know Claire). It was all pretty easy until she asked me to take small packets out from the lowest shelf in the refrigerator and put them back in. I cheated; when she said to put them back I just threw them into the boxes. Miriam said that it was "OK to use gravity to help". Occupational therapy is about thinking smart and using whatever you can, as much as it is about training the muscles to work the way they used to.

She then asked me to walk to a table in the dining room, and she made me do repeated leg squats with my left knee. After this she asked me to retrieve items from the various compartments in the cupboards in the break room while standing up unsupported, and as I did, I noticed that their inventory system was completely messed up. They had the same stuff stored in multiple locations, and where things were stored didn't match the labels on the drawers and cupboard doors. This was an affront to my years of inventory management experience, so I decided to re-organize the cupboards consolidating like items into the same boxes, grouping similar items together, taking out empty boxes, breaking them down and putting them in the recycle bin, and removing the trash etc. After 30 minutes the place was organized to my complete satisfaction, and while I wondered how long it would stay that organized, it was fun!

Back in my room, Claire finished reading the book aloud, and after lunch we had another rest on the bed, after which we got adventurous and I walked with the walker all around the unit, while Claire followed behind me with a wheelchair just in case I needed it. We went into the activity room to play Scrabble, Rummikub, and Cribbage, but it was clear that these games were not really used by people who cared. There were 200 letters in the scrabble box, no black tiles in the Rummikub box, and no pegs for the cribbage board, so we decided to rectify this situation as soon as we could get to a store, and donate some materials to the unit. This was also my last day on steroids, so I could see my dream of winning the yellow jersey in the Tour de France slipping from my grasp. My mother-in-law asked me if I could now play baseball, since I had imbibed so many steroids, and I told her that I could, just as well as I had before. She was not impressed.

Day 28

My nurse, Olivia, told me that her husband had had transverse myelitis four years before, and had made an almost complete recovery. Claire and I were incredibly interested in the exact details of his recovery, and we bombarded her with questions. She was very eager to talk with us, and answered all our questions, even the touchy ones, and she told us that she had given birth about 18 months prior, so that was very good news for us, except that we were more interested in the recreational aspects of the process, not the continuance of the species.

She brought me the scale, and after I had showered and dressed, I checked to see how much I weighed. My weight after my bladder was emptied was 168.4 pounds; not quite a healthy weight. I have never really agreed with Wendy (our Wii Fit) because she is so judgmental! She tells me "That's OVERWEIGHT" when I am 178 pounds (I am 5'11" tall). I complained about her to my doctor once, and he told me that his Wii Fit told him he was obese. I hadn't seen many men more fit than he was, so I stopped setting unrealistic weight reduction goals based on a generalized statement that all healthy adults should have a body mass index of 22. This is clearly not true. I had heard of people dropping dead at the gym from a heart attack, while working hard to reach unrealistic goals, and I was not going to be one of them. I couldn't wait to get home to tell Wendy that I finally reached her goal, by contracting a spinal cord disorder and being hospitalized for 30 days. Great planning! I had lost 10 pounds, but it didn't seem healthy, because most of the weight I lost was muscle, and I knew how difficult it would be to build it back.

Managing things like personal grooming came under the heading of OT, so Charlie, one of the other Occupational therapists helped me figure out which grooming tasks I could do standing, and which ones I might need to do sitting. As a result Claire and I recognized that we needed at least two chairs with arms on them, so that I could push myself up from the chair by using my upper body strength on the arms. I would need to do this to move from the chair to the walker and back again. Charlie also alerted us that I would need to have my feet and legs inspected daily, since I had no sensation in them and could easily injure myself without even knowing it.

Claire called our wonderful neighbors Will and Laura and asked them to find us armchairs, one for the kitchen and one to replace my rolling chair in the office, and they were thrilled to have something helpful to do. This was often the case; everyone was hungry for something to do to be helpful, and we were so grateful. We did have a list of things we had figured out that required action, so we parceled them out to different people. Of course the first thing was getting our car out of hock from the airport parking lot, and our daughter and her husband took care of that right away. Our neighbors collected our mail and sent the important stuff to us every other week or so, and they ensured that our lawn was mowed, and now took on the task of going out hunting and searching for just the right chairs. Our son was working up plans to build a ramp for the front door, and our other good friends put a bed from their house in our living room (in case I was unable to get up the stairs to sleep in our own bed) and kept the chlorinator in our pool full. Yet another friend bolted our banisters more securely to the walls so that I could actually lean on them when I did go upstairs. There were a lot of things that we needed done, and we were so thankful that we had good friends and family to do it all.

Anita, yet another Occupational therapist took me down to the activity room on the ground floor, and once again I walked the entire distance there and back with my walker. In the activity room, she challenged me with exercises to strengthen my hips and my core abdominal muscles, and I discovered that while I was in no shape to do any push-ups, I did manage to walk 10 feet across the room with no support. In the meantime, Claire went to speak with Jasmine, the clinic Case Manager, who would be putting together our discharge plan, and came back with great information.

She told me that when it came time for me to be discharged, there would be three parts to the discharge plan. First, we would have a month's supply of all the medications I would require, and we needed an appointment with Dr. Lawrence (my fun general practitioner), who would have to write new prescriptions for all my medications since a prescription written by a doctor in California would generally not be valid in New Hampshire. I would also need a prescription for an evaluation and then follow up by a Physical therapist, and so for that, I would need an appointment with my neurologist at home, Dr. Winters. Finally, I would need equipment; whatever equipment was prescribed needed to be delivered to us here in California before we left so that we could take it on the plane when we returned home. The coolest thing about this conversation was that it made real the idea that I would be going home, and in the not terribly distant future!

Claire called all my doctors to let them know what was happening with me, and to request the referral for physical therapy so that it would be approved before we got home. The bottom line was that it was a combination of Jasmine's job and our job to see that all was in place when I was discharged, and it was really nice to be talking about discharge. When we looked back at the diary we were keeping, we saw that early in the ordeal we had believed that I would be 6-9 months in a wheelchair, and here we were, thinking that we wouldn't even need to add a ramp to our front door.

When Karen came by for physical therapy we asked her who would decide when I was going to be discharged. She told us that it was a combination of what the insurance company was willing to continue to pay for, and what the staff of the rehabilitation center believed they could continue to do to improve my abilities and skills, and she told us that they were estimating two weeks! This was terrific news! We could begin to plan our homecoming! That meant August 31st would be going home day! Whoo hoo!!!

By the time her session with me was over, she had cleared me to walk independently through the unit with my walker which was multiple steps in the right direction! I spent the remainder of the PT time walking with her all around the unit with a cane, trying to look like House, but I wasn't fooling anyone even though I had the scruffy beard.

I also had a visit from an acupuncturist, who came by to tell me that it was recommended as a part of my therapy to have acupuncture, so we agreed to schedule my pincushion time for Friday, but I demanded that he only stick needles in the parts of my body that couldn't feel them!

My favorite part of the day was when Karen and I went back to the outpatient gym and I spent 15 minutes on the reclining bike with no blood pressure problems and a reasonable heart rate. It was awesome! My regular routine at home included biking as well as time on the treadmill and swimming, and here I was, back to 1/3 of my regular routine! I then conquered their terrain walkways, walkways made of different materials such as cobblestones, pine bark mulch, sand and slippery marble to train patients how to manage them. I used my walker to walk up a hill, and then wheeled my wheelchair up an inclined ramp. All of this was to prepare me for a series of scheduled outings designed to ensure that I was capable of managing in the "real world". The first was to take place the next day, when I was scheduled to go to a local grocery store to buy the ingredients to make English scones in the kitchen.

Dr. Wong, another doctor on the unit, came to talk with me in the evening about my bladder control issues, and we agreed that he would keep me on Flowmax. The alternative, to take me off the medication, might mean that I would need to go back to catheterization, and I really didn't want that again so I also agreed that I would try to remember to go to the bathroom every couple of hours so that my bladder muscle would relearn its true function.

I really had to give the staff a lot of credit. They left no stone unturned in their effort to ensure that I was prepared for independent living. While I had Claire to do the cooking, cleaning, driving, and anything else I needed help with (and I am not saying any of this in a sexist mode, but in an "eternally grateful that I have a loving wife who is retired from a full time career and enjoying being a homemaker again" attitude of gratitude) I know that there were many other patients who didn't have that luxury, so planning ahead for all of these issues was critical.

Day 29

Dmitri, yet another Occupational therapist took me into the kitchen so that I could check the cooking supplies and make sure that I had everything I needed to bake my scones. The therapy consisted of standing, unlocking and checking all the kitchen cupboards, finding the right items and placing them in an empty cupboard, placing a "do not touch" sign on them, and making sure that all was ready for baking day, which was set for three days from then. PT included walking downstairs using only a cane, and then stepping up two 14 inch stairs to simulate getting on the train, something I would need to do to get to the grocery store. This I completed successfully twice in a row, using the railing to assist me. I also spent 10 minutes using the leg press in the gym, and I was really disappointed when I could only push 30 lbs of weight compare with a previous best of 300 pounds, but my leg movements were slow and controlled, so it was a good exercise.

After lunch and a short nap, Karen and Miriam arrived for our first big outdoor adventure! While Claire followed pushing the wheelchair just in case I needed it to rest, I used my walker to walk out of the hospital, down the hill and across the street to the train stop, and we boarded the train which took us all down the hill two stops, to the Safeway grocery store. I did well getting on and off the train, and crossing the road which was criss-crossed with train tracks. At the store I gave up my walker for a grocery cart, using it for a walker, and went up and down the aisles looking for the ingredients I needed to make the scones. I also managed to pick up a few essential medical supplies, M&M's and Gummy Bears, for late night medical emergencies!

Halfway through the shopping trip I got a 15 second "restroom alert" warning; this was basically all I the warning I had at this point in my recovery before I needed to be in the bathroom voiding! My hope was that this would continue to improve, however in the meantime, I was appropriately garbed to avoid any potential "accidents". This was the first time in my life that I didn't feel guilty about using the disabled section of a public restroom. After the bathroom emergency was over I completed my shopping tasks and used the self checkout stand to scan and pay for my purchases, and then we agreed to try to walk back to the hospital, which included a quarter mile that was up a fairly steep San Francisco hill.

This hill was similar to the incline on our road at home, so I thought it would be good practice if I ever wanted to join the neighborhood walking club. I walked up the hill using the walker and only stopped once for brief rest in the wheelchair. It was a very successful shopping trip, and Claire uploaded photos to Facebook and we received many supportive comments from our friends and family, many of whom wondered how I lucked out being surrounded by beautiful women all the time!

Thanks to the internet we also discovered yet another book written by someone with TM: "The Best Seat in the House" by Allen Rucker, who was a Hollywood screen writer who had been struck by Transverse Myelitis 9 years prior to writing his book. Claire began reading it aloud, and while it was quite humorous in parts, we were sad to read that his recovery was not as far along as mine, and he was still in a wheelchair.

Day 30

The good news this morning was that I had a successful bowel program, and it killed two birds with one bullet so to speak. In this case the bullet was a 357 caliber white shell (suppository) shot at close range into the anal cavity. The impact of the bullet was felt almost immediately, and pretty soon the bowel and bladder were emptying at a good rate. This bullet pre-empted the morning bladder catheter which was required because the bladder showed 650 ml, but after the bowel program the scan said 278ml, and this was the lowest bladder scan reading at 6:00 am ever! This also meant that no catheter was needed. The whole process took less than 15 minutes to complete, so this was a very good start to the day.

Ciara (the Recreation Therapist) and Miriam came to my room at around 8:20 am to take me out for our second experimental outing: breakfast, with another patient, James, a man who was recovering from a motorcycle accident. Going on outings like this are all a part of the rehabilitation effort to get patients back to normal living. James had sustained several broken bones in the accident and was walking with a cane. Miriam decided not to take the wheelchair based on my proven ability from the day before to walk considerable distances using only a walker, and so we went down to the train stop to take the train the other direction, towards Claire's hotel. During the 15 minute wait for the train I was standing, and since we used the wheelchair ramp to get onto the train, James and I were able to sit as we rode the one stop through the tunnel. From where we got off, it was a one block walk to the restaurant where Claire was there to meet us. The crepes were great and we relished every mouthful, especially after so many days of institutionally programmed menus.

After breakfast we had to make our way across the street and over all the train tracks, and the walker from the rehab center had small hard plastic wheels which kept getting stuck in the tracks, so as I crossed the road I got frustrated with it, and I picked it up and carried it across the street. On the other side we waited another 15 minutes for a train, and when it arrived it was packed. I pulled myself up into the train as Miriam and Ciara helped James up the steps. Despite our clear disabilities, both James and I had to stand the whole way back through the tunnel, hanging on to a strap above our heads.

I looked at the occupants in the disabled seats, and mentally created a disability chart in my mind that could help separate the slightly disabled from the severely challenged. I think such a chart might become very important as aging baby boomers hit retirement and they all want the same disabled parking spot closest to their favorite restaurant.

Once back at the rehab center I took a short rest, and Claire went off for a couple of hours to try to find some blackcurrant jam (the ONLY kind to eat with scones) and a "fanny pack" so that I could carry some needed things around with me as I was out and about. While she was gone I had yet another PT session during which I walked up and down stairs with a cane and up and down the corridor several times without using it at all. By the time it was over, my legs were exhausted. After lunch, when Karen showed up for my afternoon PT session, she overrode my protestations that my legs were tired. "A lame excuse", she said, but she did allow me to take my wheelchair down to the gym where she had me work all the muscles that were not exhausted. After PT I had three satisfying minutes of complete bed rest before OT showed up.

For OT I asked to see if I could get into and out of a bathtub safely. Claire and I have a "two person" Jacuzzi tub in our bathroom, and Claire was anxious for us to get to enjoy it again, even though I reminded her that I wouldn't be able to feel the warm water in either the Jacuzzi or our hot tub! The attempt to get into the clinic tub taught me how to use my other senses to compensate for the loss of sensation in my legs, but the end result of the bathtub exercise was that it was probably more risky to try and use the bathtub than a sit down shower, and it put us on notice that we would need grab rails installed to enable me to get in and out of the shower safely.

I was finally free to rest at around 4:00 pm, just as Claire finally returned from her lengthy and fruitless shopping expedition. After trying six stores, she found no blackcurrant jam, and no fanny pack, but did find a sling that she thought would work for me, and didn't look too "girlish". Yes, I am a new age sensitive guy, but I draw the line at a man purse!

In the evening, I was in for yet another new and unique experience. Claire had scheduled me for a "remote healing session" with our Church healing team, so she sat by the door to ensure that no one would disturb me while I relaxed in my bed. Our church healing team was assembled at our home church in New Hampshire, nearly 3000 miles away, and they attempted a long distance healing. I fell totally asleep, surrounded by the prayers of our faithful healing team, and at 6:00 pm Claire, knowing by prior arrangement that the session would be over, came in and brought me my dinner. I felt remarkably refreshed, and a later report from the healing team was that they had felt as though I was right there with them, but they all felt that they had to coax my spirit back into my body.

Day 31

The day didn't start well. I woke up in the middle of the night (3:00 am) and had difficulty getting to the toilet and back to bed. My legs were wobbly and un-coordinated, and at 5:00 am I was sweating, yet I didn't seem to have a fever. The feeling disappeared after about 30 minutes, and then when my nurse Sean came in for the morning vital sign checks everything seemed in order. He wheeled in the scale, and just as I tried to stand on it, my knees gave way beneath me, and I had to use my hands to prevent a fall. Sean made a note of this in my chart. It was not classified as a fall, because at no point did I hit the ground, but I was now very unsure of my capabilities and decided to take the cautious approach. I decided to forego my usual morning shower thinking that it wouldn't be a good idea given my current weakened condition, but I did dress and try to figure out how I was going to get through the day's plan for PT and OT. When Claire arrived I told her the worrying news, and when Miriam arrived for OT, she had already read the chart, so she knew that something was wrong. She asked me if I felt up to doing some work in the kitchen, and I told her yes, so after a couple of successful knee bend and standing leg exercises, I used my walker to go to the kitchen, and I stood up while I unloaded the dishwasher and put everything away in the place that I thought it really should have been put in the first place.

I teach 5S programs at work. 5S is the name of a workplace organization methodology that describes how items are stored and maintained, and it involves sorting, straightening, systematic cleaning, standardizing, and sustaining. As a result I am convinced that I can reorganize everyone else's space far better than they can organize it themselves, so this was fun! I went with Miriam back to the room so that she could test my strength to compare today's results with her previous evaluation, and surprisingly she found that I had pretty much the same level of strength as I had several days prior, but because of how weak I was feeling, she called a halt to the OT session, and pretty soon Dr. Matthews came in to examine me. He decided that there had been a relapse, and ordered a new MRI. Two thoracic spine MRI's were completed one with contrast and one without, and in the meantime Dr. Matthews called my neurologist, Dr. Graham and they agreed to transfer me back to the hospital for a second round of plasmapheresis. They also agreed that I should be put back on intravenous steroids, so that was started.

My transfer back to the hospital was scheduled for 4:u this time GIC approval was nearly immediate, in part precipitated by Claire's urgent phone call to the Insuranc Manager at 11:00 am. Karen, Miriam and Ciara came by at .ɔ pm, all very sorry that my rehabilitation had been interrupted again, and Ciara was particularly disappointed that I wouldn't get to bake the scones, but Claire and I assured her that we would be back, and that the scones would be baked! Claire packed up my things and took most of them back to her hotel, leaving the things I would need in the hospital packed in a suitcase so that the ambulance people could transfer it with me. I was heading backwards again.

Claire wondered that she didn't fall apart during all of this drama! My recovery was occurring so fast that we had to invent new plans every day, and then, just when we felt like we were headed for the finish line, this new development came along to fling us backwards. Our emotions were in turmoil, as we were both elated (by my phenomenal recovery) and distressed (by this rapid onset of apparent weakness). Claire knew that her job was to stay strong, and to do whatever was needed to take care of everything, and I do mean everything! Marriage is a partnership, and hopefully each member of the team remains fully able to do their part to keep things going, but our roles had clearly changed. I could be held accountable and responsible for only one thing, doing whatever I could to get better. Claire had the rest!

People tell her now that if they were ever sick, they wanted her at the hospital with them. It seemed to her that all she was doing was just what was necessary, but as I read through our diary, and edit the pages of this book, I realize that what was necessary was quite a bit. The administrative stuff was a piece of cake for her, but there was so much of it! The more difficult parts were those parts that required physical strength and endurance. She doesn't think she has much of that. She sees herself as a slightly overweight wimp, and believes that "sweating" is something horses should do, not her! Yet here she was physically hauling stuff, yet again, on crowded public transportation, and I know her knees were killing her, but she just kept popping Tylenol and Nexium, and braved her way through it. We were really ready for it all to end.

Chapter 8 - Back to the Hospital

Day 31 - Continued

When we arrived back at the hospital, the same one I had come from just a week prior, I was once again assigned to a TICU (Transitional Intensive Care Unit), but I was disappointed that it was not the same TICU that I had been in before. In exchange, I got a reasonably sized room. My first visitor was Dr. Kaitlyn: Neurologist "wannabe", so I felt assured that I wouldn't have to explain everything again! My new hospitalist knew some of my recent medical history, and I gave him a copy of my report on my allergic response to the plasmapheresis and he put it into my file. My new nurse hooked me up to my new best friends, my monitoring devices and an IV line, and I went through the details of my medical history once more.

I was very surprised, pleasantly surprised, when shortly after my arrival a young man came into the room wheeling a machine, and did a chest x-ray, right there in my bed. His departure was followed almost immediately by the arrival of a young woman with yet another rolling cart, who did an EKG, and her departure was followed nearly instantaneously by the lab technician who drew my blood. It was incredible! It was like they had already read this book! Bringing health care to the patient! What a concept!

We got on Skype with our son and grandchildren who were very pleased to have a chance to see and talk to their Bampa, as they had been worried when they heard that I was going back to the hospital again. Suddenly Claire realized that my suitcase wasn't in the room. It had left the ward with me, one of the EMTs had pulled it behind her as she helped wheel me down to the transport, but Claire had to take the last of our things to her hotel before she came to the hospital, so neither of us realized that the EMT had, unfortunately, lost track of the suitcase somewhere in the process. Claire got involved with hospital security to track it down and fortunately it was located in the ambulance bay. She got it sent to where it needed to be, and we were finally reunited at about 9:15 pm.

My neurologist Dr. Graham came into the room, and due to the urgency of my transfer he was fully expecting to see me flat on my back in bed, but thanks either to the IV steroids I had been given by Dr. Mathews at rehab or to the rest I had gotten between the time everyone got "excited" and his visit, I was feeling quite well, so when he arrived, I was standing up closing my curtains. He looked quizzically at me, and said "So, what else can you do?" as he beamed like a Cheshire cat. I showed him that I could walk a few steps, and we spent about an hour discussing everything from my disorder to our favorite movies. I was very impressed by his skill level, his knowledge and his meticulous attention to detail; I was so glad that he was my neurologist. He checked my neurological functions and told me that he would consult with Dr. Hawkins, the immunologist, and they would figure out what to do next.

Interestingly, despite my weakness, Dr. Graham also told me that my newest MRI showed that considerable healing had occurred in the lesions on my spine; in fact, there was a 50% reduction in the lesions. This had occurred between July 31st, when I had my initial setback and was sent to the hospital for plasmapheresis, and August 19th, today. Once again, we were looking at a single point in time, so we didn't know how quickly the healing had occurred, exactly when it had occurred, or what had caused the improvement.

When Dr. Kaitlyn returned she did an exam and asked me to try to walk for her so that she could see what was happening with my strength and my gait. I got up from the bed, and walked unaided all the way across the room and back, and I could even stand without my knees buckling. She attributed this to massive dose of IV steroids that Dr. Matthews had put me on while still in rehab, since I hadn't gotten any other treatment, and I suggested to her that she bring up the possibility of transferring me back to the rehab center and keeping me on the steroids with another taper to see if this would work.

She told me that when the spinal tap results had come through there were a couple of markers (indicators) for MS, so she wanted to keep me in the hospital for a while so that they could check on those results. She noted our alarm when she reported these results to us, but she reminded us that it was only some of the markers, and that it certainly didn't mean that I had MS. She told us that she would be running some more panels to check on the results, and determine for certain whether or not MS was a new diagnosis.

This visit gave me a chance to ask her about the dangers of taking steroids for an extended period of time, since it appeared that with steroids I got better, and when I tapered off of them I got worse. She told me that while I had experienced a lot of success and great results with steroids, they did compromise the body's immune system, and they had serious side effects over the long term. In any event, she told me, it would ultimately be Dr. Hawkins and Dr. Graham who would decide what further treatment would be recommended. In particular, Dr. Hawkins would need to make the decision about whether or not to pursue further plasmapheresis treatments. I was grateful that he was well aware of my allergic response, and of the risks and precautions that had to be in place before and during the process.

I waited up in case the good doctors decided they wanted to stick another jugular catheter in my neck, and used my time to research the differences between TM and MS; I might not be in rehab, and I might not have a high definition flat screen TV, but I had internet without having to chase someone down!

Day 32

I woke up feeling extremely strong and I was raring to go. I had regained all the strength that I had lost the previous day, and I may even have gained some more, so I got up and decided to measure my strength. I stood unsupported by the side of the bed for 5 full minutes, completely balanced; just 24 hours after my knees had buckled beneath me just getting on the scale.

The doctors came in to examine me and most of them were new to me. This was a new team, headed by Dr. White whom we had met before, once, while in the ICU. One of the young doctors with Dr. White came from Nashua, New Hampshire, and she was keen to talk with me and find out all about why I was here. Shortly after my group interview, one of the doctors came back and asked me to walk across the room. She couldn't have weighed more than 100 pounds, so I warned her that I was a fall risk, and she told me that she understood. I managed to walk to the door of the room and back without falling or having my knees buckle and without knocking her out the window.

The standard "you get what we give you because we didn't bother asking you for your preferences" breakfast was served at 8:45 am. This is what happens when you move faster than the hospital does. The system only worked if you were there the day before; it was quite a dysfunctional system.

The new team of doctors doing rounds came by at 10:30 am and after discussing what little they knew, left us waiting to hear from Dr. Hawkins. Only he could decide what to do next. Dr. White did tell us that the team would come back to insert the jugular catheter right after rounds so that we could be ready to start the plasmapheresis as soon as Dr. Hawkins gave the go ahead.

A physical therapist, John, came in at 11:00 and he brought me a walker with rubber wheels that were three times the size of the puny ones on the walker I had used in rehab. With wheels like these, I could go off road! Woohoo! I was ready to travel, but sadly my telemetry unit didn't have much range, so travel was not in the cards, but John did allow me to walk around the nurses' station a couple of times and noticed that while I started off walking with some difficulty, it quickly became easier and easier for me to walk. I told John that I was able to use the regular toilet and that I had been cleared to shower myself while I was in rehab. John finished his session by clearing me to ambulate around the room, take a shower and use the toilet on my own; I was gaining more independence daily.

The doctors didn't come back after rounds, or after lunch, and I had just woken up from a nap when the nurse put through a call from Dr. Hawkins. He apologized for not being "on the case" sooner but he took the time to explain the whole problem with any attempt at continuing plasmapheresis. Interestingly, it was a supply chain problem; just what my entire career has been about!

The primary problem was that the kind of allergic reaction that I had experienced happened so infrequently that the hospital supply chain simply couldn't accommodate it. The hospital bought their Albumin in quantity from a single supplier and they didn't have an alternate source. As a result, it could take up to two weeks to get a new supply to the pharmacy for my use, so at a minimum I would be sitting around for two weeks waiting for a new supply of Albumin to be delivered. I was by no means assured that the quoted two week lead time was accurate, and I was absolutely not interested in wasting two weeks waiting for some delivery truck to show up, so we agreed that plasmapheresis was out of the question.

Buying in bulk, buying at the best value, and developing partnerships between suppliers and customers are critical to an efficient and cost effective system, but when patients' lives and well being are on the line, the system must also be sufficiently flexible to allow the ability to get required products immediately. Today, as a consumer, I can go on line and get nearly anything I want delivered to my home within 48 hours (assuming that it exists). There isn't one reason I can think of why a hospital supply system shouldn't be able to get five bottles of Albumin from a different manufacturer within the same period of time.

Systems are there to help facilitate the process, but they very quickly become the process, and people fail to look outside the box. If there was ever a system which required people to constantly look outside the box, it is the medical system.

Interestingly, Dr. Hawkins didn't actually think that it was my best treatment option at this point anyway, given that I had responded so well to the steroids; after all, I had regained all of my lost strength in less than 12 hours.

He believed that most of the reduction in the lesions had been the result of the steroids, not the plasmapheresis; his estimate was 75% steroids, 25% plasmapheresis. He had discussed this with Dr. Graham and they had agreed, so they decided to transfer me to a regular ward, continue the steroids (oral now, not IV) but this time they wanted to taper me off the steroids over several weeks, not days. In hindsight (always 20/20) it was at this moment, on this Friday, in the afternoon before the business offices closed, that Claire should have called the GIC case manager and asked for her to expedite my transfer back to rehab, but we talked about it, and we agreed (me, reluctantly) that I was doing well, that we could do a lot on our own, and that it was not an emergency, so we would allow the system do its "thing" (its "thing" was Friday afternoon to Tuesday afternoon, four days).

The previous two times I had been on steroids I had tapered off over several days, decreasing from 60 mg of Prednisone to nothing by 10 mg a day the first time, and by 5 mg a day the second time. Now they were talking 30 days. I agreed with this approach since it avoided the risks and delays associated with continuing plasmapheresis, and it increased the chances for going home sooner, which had now become everyone's goal. The bad news was, that as we looked ahead to what was in our schedule, and if all went well, and if I was able to teach the classes that had been rescheduled from July and August into September, the taper would end while I was still in California, and Claire was adamant that I not go off the steroids until I was home. Don't get me wrong, she loved California, but she did not want to LIVE here, and especially not in a small hotel room traveling 90 minutes each way to come see me every day. She was insistent that whatever the plan, I not go off my steroids one second earlier than the plane landing in Boston. Dr. Hawkins didn't see any problem with this, but as it happens, others did, so Claire had another mission. She would ensure that I had enough steroids to take me all the way home, even if she had to steal them!

Susan (the wonderful physical therapist I had seen so many times when I had been here before) stopped in as she was leaving to go home, and it was great to see her again. She had kept in touch with Karen (with our permission), the therapist from rehab, and had heard about all the outings that we had gone on during the week, and promised to drop in again. She assured us that I was a high priority patient for PT the next day (Saturday) though she did tell me that there would be no therapists working on Sunday.

After dinner was delivered, Claire left for her bus trip back to her hotel, now, once again, having a 90 minute journey back, and Dr. Graham came by and told me that I would be transferred to another ward since I didn't require telemetry anymore. Since Claire had gone, I got to pack my things myself and get myself ready for the transfer.

Perhaps there was another patient in urgent need of my TICU bed, I had no way of knowing, so maybe my transfer out of the TICU to a regular ward at 11:00 pm was justified, but given my capability I had a very difficult time getting my things packed to move.

The staff came to move me at 11:00 pm, took me to another ward, and attempted to move me into a small room in which there already was a patient. From the outside of the room I could see that it was the smallest room I had seen thus far in the hospital, with a curtain that divided it down the middle making it even smaller than Claire's little hotel room. It had space for a bed, and very little else. I explained that I had a wheelchair and a walker in addition to my suitcase, and that there was clearly insufficient room for me and my equipment in this space. The staff went to their magic whiteboard, and reluctantly did some room shuffling, and while they were figuring out what to do, I chatted with Tabitha, who along with Kaitlyn, Carla and Kat had made up the Dream Team that treated me during my previous visit. She told me that she would be a part of the team taking care of me while I was on this ward, and I was thrilled. There is nothing like knowing the people caring for you when you are trying to get better!

In the meantime, the charge nurse decided to put me into a much larger room on my own. Unfortunately for the patient currently in that room, it meant that he had to move out of that huge space into another room, and I didn't ask, and didn't want to know where that was! I thought that it was unconscionable that they made the patient in that room move at 11:00 pm. A little thought, a few minutes of consideration would have revealed numerous alternatives which would have allowed both of us to have more rest. For example, my suitcase could have been put in my room, but the wheelchair left in the hall until the morning, after all, I didn't need it to go to the bathroom, my walker was sufficient, and even if that were it an issue, I could have had a condom catheter put on so that at least, for that night, I wouldn't have had to get up out of bed to go to the bathroom. But move him they did, and I was going to have lots of room for me, my wife, and my equipment.

I unpacked my stuff and put it all away in the closet and drawers, and the staff gradually brought me all the things that I needed. I took advantage of the opportunity to turn off the television that was blaring at me from the other half of the room. Housekeeping came in to clean it, and my nurse who came in to do the initial nursing assessment told me that unless they needed the space, I would have the room to myself. I told her that I needed a bladder scan and she was very impressed; she didn't normally have such well informed patients. By the time everything was done it was 1:00 am; my nurse said "enjoy your sleep, they will be in at 5:00 am to draw your blood" and turned out the lights.

Day 33

I woke up at 4:50 am, just before the expected vampire, and my nurse came in shortly after my blood was drawn, and my bladder scan indicated 440 ml, so everything was flowing the

153

way it should be, and I didn't need to be catheterized. Claire and I had agreed that since we were not in rehab any longer, we had to take charge of our own PT program, so we agreed to four periods of PT a day. I stared with a shower! Here I discovered yet another of the interesting things about the supply system. Up until now, I had been given what I needed for my shower ready to use, but in this case, I got a small travel sized bottle of shampoo which had not been opened, and which, I discovered was impossible to open without a very sharp implement. It became obvious to me that the people who ordered the stuff never had to use it, but despite that, once I broke into it with my pen, I had a great shower!

It is amazing what a difference it makes to have a shower! I navigated my walker sideways (that was the only way it would fit) into the shower, two legs at a time, stepping into the shower myself after the first two walker legs were inside. It took a while to adjust the water temperature correctly, since cold water felt warm on my legs, and scalding hot water felt cool on my legs. As a result, I had to be VERY careful with things like that!

When Dr. Tabitha came in for a chat we talked about the steroid taper, as well as the quantity of steroid I was getting. We were very fixed on the Prednisone taper and on making sure that I would take my last pill the day we went home to New Hampshire, so that if I did have a relapse again it would be in NH. Dr. Graham was reluctant to have the taper be more than 30 days, which put us back in California again. I knew my wife wouldn't stand for this; she would find a way to make it work to her satisfaction, even if she had to sequester pills out of the stash I would be given to prolong the taper.

Following Tabitha's visit, Claire and I started on my PT with the therabands and exercises in bed, and while I was doing my exercises, a Physical therapist came in. She took me directly to do stairs, which surprised us, even though it was one of the things that most concerned us about my ability once we got home. She asked me how many stairs I had at home, and I did a quick count in my head and came up with 56. She was quite surprised and asked why we had so many, so I explained that we lived in a four story house on a hill, and that there were three regular flights of 14 stairs, plus a spiral staircase of 14 stairs into our pool building. She realized that stairs were a big deal for me!

Claire followed us, as the therapist took me to the hospital exit stairwell down the hall, and I went up seven stairs to the landing, and then up another seven steps, and then came down the same 14 steps. Then I walked, without the walker down the long hallway back to my room. Once back in my room, she put me through more exercises standing, in a chair, and lying down; she could have matched Greg for her intensity in seeing to it that I could "be all that I could be". She was quite the taskmaster! When she left, Claire and I looked at each other and smiled. I had done so much, and we were both very pleased!

Following all that work, we continued reading the second book (Allen Rucker's "Best Seat in the House") and later, with Claire's help, I walked all around the floor of the hospital for about 30 minutes, without stopping! It was quite an achievement!

We talked about what type of equipment we should order for both home and work. We agreed that it didn't look like we would need a wheelchair in the house, but that we should probably get one to take with us on local trips in the car at home, and should keep one in California for when we teach, so we looked on the internet at what was "out there" and made some decisions.

Day 34

I was astounded to wake up after a full 6 hours of uninterrupted sleep, and when my nurse came in at 6:00 am, she asked me not to take a shower because it was shift change and she wanted to introduce me to my new nurse, and so when Claire came in at 7:10 am, she found me very frustrated. We waited until 7:40 am for the turnover introductions, and when my new nurse asked if there was anything that I needed, I told her that I would really like to take a shower, but she told me that I couldn't have one, because the IV lines weren't covered. They had never been covered before, so when she hadn't returned to cover my IV lines by 8:15 am Claire and I took matters into our own hands. Claire went out in the hall and got towels and floor mats from the linen cart, and I took a shower anyway.

Claire had brought me some clothes to wear, so I got dressed and I had just started to eat my breakfast when another of our "Dream Team" docs arrived. This was Doctor Carla, and she was delighted to learn of my continued rapid recovery, and was even more amazed when she performed her neurological tests and saw how far I had progressed in my abilities. My sensation, however, hadn't changed at all, and while she didn't say anything about that, it was a concern to Claire and me.

Karson, Sharon's husband and our good friend from our 2000 trip to China had arranged to come for a visit. We checked to make sure that we had permission to leave the unit, and when he arrived we went down to the cafeteria and spent a very pleasant couple of hours with him. I walked down to the cafeteria with my walker and he was very impressed with my improvement, since he had heard from his wife after her visit, that I was bedridden. As I mentioned earlier, Karson is the current President of the professional society to which both

Claire and I belong and of which I was a former president. He was returning from a local meeting and was on his way home. We talked about my health of course, but it was truly great when we talked at length about the state of the professional association, as well as his health and his future plans after he was no longer someone who was important. It was just nice to talk about something other than my health; it was a delightful visit!

After lunch, PT, more exercises and some pleasant cuddle time, Claire prepared a snack of cheese and crackers, an idea she had gotten when some friends sent us a box of fruit, cheese and crackers. From then on, on weekends, we had a special snack, and it was a real treat (which would have been a lot better with red wine!) Claire carried on reading "Best Seat in the House", we played some cribbage and I did quite a bit of standing.

Day 35

I was a horribly impatient patient and now my patience was being taxed to the max. I was ready to go back to rehab; a decision had been made to transfer me back to rehab, and now it was time to implement it, so when I woke up I was anxious to get things moving with the transfer. After breakfast I checked with the nurse to see what was happening and she told me that the hospital case manager wasn't in her office yet, that she normally came in at 9:30 am, and that it was her job to get everything in line for my transfer.

I spent the time wisely. While still at rehab, we had talked with Karen and Miriam about a "home" visit. Since my home was nearly 3000 miles away, we decided to go to my client's to see the training set up, the restroom facilities, and to go to the hotel we called "home" while working and check out their disabled rooms, so I called Silena, my client contact, to see if we could do this, and she was very glad to hear from me. She welcomed the idea of a visit, and told me when the training room was available. Armed with this information, Claire called the hotel and spoke directly with the manager, who said he would be more than happy to let us come visit and see the rooms that they had for handicapped people so that we could pick whichever one we wanted and ask for it when we made our reservation.

Claire and I used the time to finish reading Allen Rucker's book; Claire read the book while I did my exercises, and then another physical therapist came by to put me through more exercises. This time I walked up and down two flights of stairs, walked unaided down the corridor several times, I stepped up on a step stool which suddenly didn't seem quite as much of an obstacle anymore, and completed every exercise that the therapist came up with. She admitted that I was a bit of a problem, because she was running out of things to challenge me with.

Lunch came and went with no transfer information accompaniment, and when Dr. Varney came by we complained about the delay. He just held up his hands and told us that he had nothing to do with that. It was extremely frustrating when something needed to happen and no one was willing to take responsibility for making it so; when people all pointed in another direction and said "It is not my job". If we want the health care system to work, it must act as one system, with everyone accepting responsibility for making it act as one system. That includes the doctors. The bureaucracy is a part of the problem; it has become so complicated that no one can negotiate it quickly enough to make it work effectively. It must become more seamless, and that means breaking down the barriers.

W. Edwards Deming, the original Total Quality Guru wrote 14 rules for implementing quality, and one of them was "Break down barriers between departments" and in this case, it would be better to say between "institutions". Communication must be instantaneous, analysis and review must be ongoing, and the focus must be on what is the best action, in this minute, for the patient. In addition, this must occur 24 hours a day up to 366 days a year (I am very sensitive about this point, since I am a leap year baby).

No one should ever say "it isn't my job" or "I can't do anything about that". If it has to do with patient care, it is your job, and if you can't do something about it then you make it your responsibility to find someone who can. So we spent the frustrating time in the afternoon working on preparing for the next course we were teaching in September and continuing the work on preparing to teach the new course that we were scheduled to teach twice in September.

When the case manager, Madge, finally came in, she told us that the transfer request was in the hands of GIC and that they were working on it. What this meant was that the clock that the insurance company used to track their work, 24 to 48 hours to get the transfer processed, had now been ticking since noon Monday, whereas the ball could have started rolling on Friday afternoon when the decision to transfer had been made by the hospital. The whole process is ridiculous, and it has nothing to do with the best interests of the patient; it is all about following some bureaucratic process. Time kept on ticking away; it approached Madge's quitting time so it was clear that we were not going to be going anywhere soon, so Claire went to California Pizza Kitchen to buy us a special dinner! It tasted really terrific after the bland hospital fare.

Tabitha from the "Dream Team" came by to tell me that Dr. Graham had approved the 40 day taper for the Prednisone, and that was highly reassuring, since it meant that Claire didn't have to resort to criminal activity to ensure that I was home when I came off the steroids. Then at about 8:30 pm, after Claire had gone, I got a roommate.

I knew that I had been really lucky to have this enormous room all to myself for this long, so I moved everything, wheelchair, suitcase, walker, tables, etc., all into my half of the room. My roommate arrived, and talked incessantly and very loudly with the nurses, doctors and staff, and he kept his light on and his TV on all night. Apparently he didn't sleep much at night, so I knew that I wouldn't be getting much rest while he was in my room. It is amazing how contradictory hospitals can be, on one hand they make a big deal about privacy, they put up signs in elevators to stop you talking about patients, but then they cram you in a room with a curtain divider and everything you hear is a privacy violation. I didn't need to know the exact details of his medical condition, and I am sure he wasn't interested in mine. I was now even more determined to leave quickly.

Day 36

I finally got some sleep, roughly three and a half hours, and had showered, dressed and breakfasted, met with the doctor, been to the cafeteria for a good coffee, and was continuing working on my exercises, when it was PT time and I asked to repeat the balance and strength tests that Karen had given me in rehab. Then I had scored a 37, but this time I managed to score 49 out of 56 on the test, a great improvement in 11 days. I was delighted with my progress, and began developing an escape plan.

Based on the results I had just achieved I believed I was capable of independent living, and didn't even need to go back to rehab, so I figured if we didn't hear from the insurance company by the end of the day, I would just request a discharge, check into a hotel for the night and fly home the next day. When I discussed this plan with Claire, she agreed in principle (while not in the details) and so she called the airline, and made our reservation for the night flight on the 29th. On August 30th we would be home.

The medical system had brought us such a long way, but we felt a level of confidence that we could continue the journey without hospitals. We knew the future wasn't going to be as easy or as comfortable as the life we had before TM, but we also knew that we were resourceful, and would be able to get what we needed to ensure that I remained strong and healthy. We were just tired of the hospital food, atmosphere, bureaucracy, emotional sterility, and wanted our independence back, and this included the comfort of our own house, our family and our friends.

We were extremely lucky that we were able to emotionally connect with a good number of the medical professionals we encountered, while not on a deep level, at least on a personal level. Claire had two major hospital experiences, each of which was about this same length of time, and in each case, numbness, depression and lethargy had resulted, in part from the lack of emotional stimulation. At least Claire and I had each other, and had developed some personal relationships with staff, but it was still bad enough that we were ready to try it our way.

After PT Claire and I continued to work on preparing to teach a new course which was a very productive use of our time. Every couple of hours we would break and continue my workouts, and occasionally Madge, the hospital case manager, came by to tell us that she hadn't heard anything yet. After lunch I took a short nap, trying to catch up on my lack of sleep from the night before, and at about 2:30 pm I got a phone call from Rosie, the patient with TM we had connected with on my previous visit. We had found out that she was no longer a patient when we came back to the hospital, so it was great to hear that she was doing well at home with physical therapy, but I continued to try to talk her into a concentrated rehabilitation program like the one I had been in. We ended our call when both Madge and Dr. Varney came in to tell us that the transfer to rehab had been approved, was scheduled for 4:00 pm, so we packed quickly, grinning like kids, and got ourselves ready to leave. We had no regrets; this was the best answer that we could think of, giving us a few more days for recovery and time to set up the things we still needed to take care of before going home.

We wondered, even in our excitement about having a date to go home, that the whole process of executing transfers from hospital to rehab, from rehab to hospital, and back and forth again didn't threaten my health. Additionally, we were sure that the total cost of my care included huge quantities of waste, which in our case, ultimately would be paid for by the taxpayer, since our insurance is government funded. It seemed to us that if the insurance company had an empowered employee on call, to make and execute decisions about transfers during non-working hours, the entire system could save many times that person's salary in costs.

At present, we have no idea what the final cost of the entire hospitalization and rehabilitation will be, either for us or for the insurance company, but we do know that there were days for which someone was paying, and during which no real treatment was taking place because we were in the wrong place. That is a waste to the entire system.

Chapter 9 - Back in Rehab Again

We arrived back in rehab to the smiling faces of all the people we knew, and they were clearly pleased to see us back again. We settled into our new room, which was not quite as large as our previous room, and didn't have quite as great a view as our previous room, and of course, didn't have internet service. Aaron told us that they had been working on it all week, and so there was hope, but they would probably finish the installation the day after we left, and we were scheduled to leave in five days. We just had to count down the days to our departure.

Day 37

After a restful night's sleep and having totally enjoyed the privacy and silence of my single room, my bladder scan showed my lowest reading in my limited recorded medical history. I took my first Fosamex tablet, a new requirement based on my long term steroid use, which required an empty stomach and sitting up at an angle of more than 30 degrees for 30 minutes.

As one of my clients was a pharmaceutical company, I had to wonder how they had decided on this method. I wondered how the clinical trials had been conducted, and whether they had bent patients at different angles for different periods of time, with full, partially full or empty stomachs in order to determine the best approach. It seemed that they had a lot of variables to consider to arrive at this specific determination. Now, I am not saying they made this up; I am just saying that there is a possibility that these operating instructions were pulled out of somewhere! You have time to think about things like this when you are trapped, immobile, by your medication. After I had sat, appropriately angled, for the allotted time, I requested towels, had a good shower and got dressed. My schedule was on my door in a timely manner, and I was scheduled for two occupational therapy sessions and for two physical therapy sessions.

Miriam arrived for occupational therapy, and we decided that this was the day I was going to bake the scones, so Claire went back to her hotel and gathered together all of the items we had purchased for this event, and brought them back with her. Meanwhile I walked unaided down to the gym where I met Karen, and she issued me with my own personal, brand new, lowest bidder, walker, which was of the same small wheeled design as the one that I had tried (somewhat successfully) to use on the trolley track filled streets of San Francisco. It could work inside the house, although I was worried that the small hard plastic wheels would play havoc with our hardwood flooring, so I asked about upgrading, but Karen informed me that it was standard issue.

I asked if I might get it in another color, and Karen, laughing, told me that since the silver color matched the hair color of most of those who used them, it was the only color they came in, but she reminded me that I could always go to Home Depot, pick up a can of spray paint, and paint it any color I liked. I asked if it came with any options, and Karen responded "Sure, you have the option of not taking it". We laughed, and Claire and I decided to do some on line shopping once we got internet.

Speaking of internet, as I was on my walkabout, I noticed that our previous room was vacant, so I asked Hazel, our very British charge nurse, if I could move back into my old room, which I knew had internet, and she said she didn't know why not! Claire and I gleefully spent the next half hour transitioning, and once we had internet again, we found a much better walker on line. It was dark blue, it folded neatly, it had its own seat, four

large rubber wheels, two sets of brakes, ⎯
the remarkable price of $75 including ship

Funny how insurance companies focus on c
costs, yet ignore the massive ones, like how
keep me an extra four days in the hospital, w
been in rehab, and perhaps gotten discharged

My mother always said "you get what you pay for", to which I
replied "you will always pay for what you get". Her philosophy
was based on the premise that anything of value should carry a
premium price; my philosophy was that if a sales person thinks
you are an easy mark, the price always goes up.

After getting my substandard walker, we walked back to the
kitchen, and Miriam left me there preparing the ingredients for
the scones, while she went to meet with Jasmine, the clinic case
manager, and among other things, told Jasmine of our revised
departure date. When Miriam came back, she and Jasmine had
organized the delivery of a wheelchair from a company with an
operation in Portsmouth, New Hampshire. The wheelchair
would be delivered to me at the rehab facility on Friday, and I
would be able to use it until I didn't need it anymore, and then I
could call them to come pick it up from our house. Now, that
was a user friendly plan!

Hazel organized for us to have the transitional suite on Saturday
and Sunday, before our departure, and Jasmine arranged for me
to get all the prescriptions I would need in time to get them
filled on Friday as well. A well organized plan!

All this was accomplished before 9:00 am while I was preparing
the scones, so it was a very good start for the day. While I was
in the kitchen preparing the scones, Hazel came in. One of the
reasons that I was baking the scones was as a treat for her. She

y from England, although she had been in the US
ears nursing all over the country, and I thought she
t like the treat, but I wanted it to be a surprise, so I was
glad that she was too busy to notice exactly what I was doing.

Baking the scones was easier than distributing them.
Apparently the Joint Commission has very strict rules on
Occupational therapy Kitchen Creations. Patients may prepare
whatever food they like in the kitchen, provided that they do
not consume any of it. They can serve it to their friends, family
and even the staff provided they advise everyone that they
consume it at their own risk, but the patient may not eat the
fruit of his/her labor. I guess they expect the patient to finish
up an occupational therapy session by throwing all the prepared
food away. This policy seemed completely inane, and was
obviously based on an incident when a patient became ill after
eating one of his/her own creations.

I have never, however, been one to follow policies or rules that I
don't agree with; I figure if I didn't have input into setting the
rules, then I shouldn't have to be bound by them if I disagree
with them. Fortunately there are a lot of rules and laws that I
do agree with, so I have yet to be incarcerated for my beliefs.

On reflection, the hospital rule made sense from a purely
defensive point of view; trying to protect the hospital from a
lawsuit when a patient killed themselves as a result of their own
cooking, when the family thought that the hospital should have
known better than to let a high risk rehab patient in the kitchen
with access to sharp cookie sheets and dangerous ingredients.
Nevertheless I was prepared to take the risk of eating my own
scones, as I had been for many years, so at 9:30 am Claire called
Hazel to come in, and after her delighted exclamation of
surprise, we all sat down to eat the scones. They were a big hit
with everyone who tried them, especially Hazel who was most

impressed, and I had numerous requests for my recipe, so I include it here:

Keith's Scones

Preheat the oven to 450 degrees
Ingredients for one batch of 12 scones
2 cups of flour
1 tablespoon baking powder
3 tablespoons sugar
½ teaspoon salt
8 tablespoons unsalted butter, chilled and cut into cubes
1 egg
½ cup milk
¼ cup golden raisins

Wash your hands.

Combine the flour, baking powder, sugar, and salt, and mix them well. Add the cold butter cubes and with your fingers (clean of course) work the mixture until it resembles coarse meal.

Break the egg into a small bowl and whisk it lightly. Pour half of it into a ½ cup measure and add milk to complete the ½ cup. (This is much more easily executed by making a double batch, and using one egg plus milk to make 1 cup and using the second egg (see directions below for the second egg) with 2 tablespoons of milk). Pour this over the flour mixture and combine (again with clean hands) until the dough forms a cohesive ball and no longer sticks to your hands. You may need to sprinkle on additional flour if the dough sticks to your hands. Knead in the golden raisins, and then turn it out onto a cutting board. Pat or roll it to ½ inch thick. Using a round cutter cut the dough and place the scones on a treated baking sheet or parchment paper.

Add 1 tablespoon milk to the remaining half egg (or 2 tablespoons with the second egg if making two batches), and using a pastry brush, lightly moisten the top of each scone.

Bake until the tops are golden, about 12-15 minutes. Cool for 10 minutes prior to serving. Once cooled they can be frozen, and then when microwaved for 30-45 seconds they will taste like fresh baked. Serve with clotted cream (and I defy you to find that in America) or whipped cream (if you are like most people and can't find clotted cream) and jam (preferably blackcurrant). Tea is optional. Eat.
The recipe makes 10-12 2 inch scones.

We did manage to keep three scones back for my doctors, but the rest of the double batch disappeared in a hurry.

During this experience we also got to meet several of the patients who were sufficiently ambulatory to make it around the unit on their own and down to the activity room. Several we were able to get to know something about, but one we had a bit of a worrisome experience with, teaching us yet another thing to fear in the hospital.

She was a middle aged woman who was free to ambulate in a wheelchair around the unit on her own, and while Claire was fixing some tea, the woman asked Claire to please get her a tea bag and pour her some hot water. Since the woman was wheelchair bound, Claire, not thinking anything about it, did as she asked. About 10 minutes later a nurse came in, took the cup from her, and said to her "You know you aren't allowed to have anything to drink!" Claire was appalled! She had just done something she thought was kind for someone and may have jeopardized her health! Hospitals are frightening places!

The reaction of the nurse to the fact that the patient had a cup of tea in front of her was not so dramatic as to make Claire think that she had jeopardized her life, but it was so unnecessary. A note should have been posted on her chair or on the door of the tea cupboard, or somewhere so that no one would make a mistake and facilitate her having something that was bad for her.

I was thrilled to see my nurse Olivia again; she was the nurse whose husband had TM. She brought me in some green tea that her husband used every day to ensure regular waste elimination. It was called "Ballerina Tea", and Olivia told me that if I drank it before I went to bed at night, in the morning I would be regular as clockwork. I thought it would be worth trying, but I insisted that I would NOT wear a tutu or spend all day twirling around.

I carried on with my physical therapy with Karen, and she taught me how to do some squat and balance exercises with a Swiss ball. We talked about exercises I could do at home using the equipment I already had in the fitness center, and she organized for Jessica, the physical therapist/yoga instructor, to spend some time with me on Sunday (our last day!!!) to discuss which yoga exercises I could do safely. I impressed her by how easily I could walk up and down a flight of stairs, and she did a strength assessment, and was very impressed by how good my bridging was compared with my previous ability.

I needed some skin cream so I asked the nurse for some. They didn't keep it on the unit, and when it still hadn't arrived by 5:30 pm, I knew that communication had broken down, but I didn't know where. I had no way of verifying if the order had been placed, if the product was in the stockroom, if it was on back order, if it had been delivered to the nurses' station, or if it had been delivered to the wrong patient. These were simply my excuses for why I didn't have it, me, a person with a lot of supply chain management experience operating in the information vacuum of a hospital supply system. There should be a fixed and immediate process for a patient to be able to get the consumable supplies he/she may need, whether that is toothpaste, shampoo or socks, and the patient should know what that process is. In the absence of information I waited until nothing showed up in what I considered to be "normal" lead time, so then Claire asked about it again, and got a rather curt response. Ten hours after my initial request I received two tubes. It doesn't take a supply chain expert to figure out something is seriously wrong with the supply system!

We were set up for our "home" evaluation for Thursday afternoon, and the plan was that we would take a taxi to the hotel, check out their disabled rooms, then Claire would push me in my wheelchair across the street to the training building, just as she would in September when I went back to teaching, and we would all see how well I could manage in a classroom environment.

After Dr. Mathews and his team examined me, all were in agreement that my recovery was on track, and that the extended course of steroids with the lengthier taper would solve the minor setbacks that had occurred twice already.

Once again I had fallen between the cracks in the food delivery system. I hadn't been here the day before so I didn't get to pick any food, so Claire took off using her bus pass to get me a celebratory dinner from Johnny Rockets. We were going home soon, and we didn't have to change another non-refundable, but multi-chargeable, airline ticket. Finally everything was going according to our plan, or perhaps everyone else just gave up trying to fight us and conceded.

Day 38

I got up, showered, got dressed and had breakfast, and Karen took me to the gym where she worked on exercises to improve my core muscle strength. My six pack abs had turned into a keg and needed a lot of work. She also encouraged me to do some of the exercises that I usually did at home, and was impressed as I held the plank steady and balanced for about a minute, and even managed 10 regular push-ups. Then I ascended the 8 inch riser staircase in a normal walking fashion, alternating feet on the stairs walking like a normal person!

When Miriam arrived I had a plan. I wanted to try again to get into a high sided bath tub without using a grab bar. I managed this with considerable ease. Then I wanted to go into the conference room and see if I could stand up and give a presentation. It took her a while to figure out how the presentation display system worked, but together we got it going, and I made a short presentation. I did well for about 10 minutes of high energy teaching in a standing position, but then it was obvious that I needed a rest, and I realized that I would have to be very careful of my energy level if I expected to teach a three day course in less than four weeks.

Then it was Ciara's time for recreational therapy, and I didn't know what she had in mind, until she suggested Tai Chi. I thought she said "Chai Tea", so I was somewhat surprised when we went into the activity room, and pretended that we were actors in a "Karate Kid" movie. I had no idea how much effort would be involved, and I gamely copied all the moves that Ciara demonstrated, even though I thought that I probably looked pretty silly, which was confirmed by the photos that Claire put up on Facebook that afternoon.

When the nearly three hours of therapy were over, I came back to the room, and collapsed on the bed, for a well earned nap, slept through lunch, and woke up at 1:00 to grab a bite and get ready for the "home" (hotel/company) afternoon outing and evaluation.

Miriam and Karen arrived promptly and Claire and I were ready to go. We borrowed a wheelchair from the unit since mine hadn't arrived, and also took my walker. The taxi driver took us to the hotel first, and one of our favorite staff people was on duty. She was very pleased to see me, especially standing upright and appearing to be very much like my old self. The general manager showed us around the disabled rooms, and I managed to guide my wheelchair everywhere I needed to be with no difficulty. I inspected the shower, made use of the facilities, and reported that the toilet seat was loose and should be fixed, before it converted the able bodied into the disabled.

We picked the room we preferred and made our reservation for September, and then I got in the wheelchair and Claire pushed me across the street to the building where I would be teaching. We met Silena who was delighted to see me standing up. This was a huge difference from when she had last seen me in the hospital. Then, I had been able to get around in the electric wheelchair, but now I was vertical and independently mobile. She escorted us all upstairs to the conference room, and I checked out how I could manage in the classroom while Karen and Miriam made many suggestions for how I could best safeguard my energy and take care of myself. I wanted to use a standard chair, as I had in my experimental session that morning, but the chair wouldn't roll easily on the carpeting, so it seemed that I would need to use my wheelchair after all. We talked with Silena about the room layout, and then went to the break area, and I checked out the men's restroom. I also went to the training department and saw all of my coworkers who were quite pleased to see that I looked so well.

After we had finished a successful evaluation of the occupational environment, I got back into the wheelchair and Karen pushed me back to the hotel. Since the cab company with which the hospital had a contract wouldn't pick us up at the hotel, we decided to take the hotel shuttle to the airport and find one of their company taxis there. This was my first time getting into a van like the one we had at home, and I managed to get up into the van with no difficulty, even though the shuttle had no grab bars on the doors. This was very encouraging.

Once we arrived at the airport I got to experiment with one more challenge. I went down an escalator, and then pushed an unaccompanied luggage cart along the sidewalk to the taxi stand. We took a taxi of the right variety back to the rehab center, and after posting a Facebook update and some photos from the outing we went into the dining room and had a game of Uno with two of the other patients. We exchanged stories, and they encouraged me to write a motivational book and speak about my experiences with this disorder and with the medical system.

There was strawberry rhubarb pie for dessert (pie was offered two or three times a week, usually for both lunch and dinner on the same day, and was a favorite) and Claire managed to make some English Custard which I shared with some of the other patients. It was at this time that the woman to whom Claire had given the cup of tea wheeled herself in. She was the only patient who was up and around who was still wearing her hospital gown instead of what Claire called "civilian clothes" and her gown was wide open in the back so that you could see her bare back and the upper part of her buttocks. Claire, embarrassed for her, went over and offered to close her gown for her, and did the best she could to give the woman some coverage, but it was a sad sight. She was appalled when she saw how exposed the woman was; she couldn't believe that her nurse had let her out of her room that way. She knew enough early in the game to get me two gowns, one of which was worn open in the back, and the second, like a robe, open in the front. This woman clearly should have been given two gowns and taught how to use them properly or had help dressing. Patient dignity is sufficiently depleted just by virtue of being in the hospital and having procedures done in an open or fairly open environment. Adding to this by being allowed to wander exposed was completely inappropriate.

Day 39

I had a fairly quiet morning as my first session was not until 11:00, and the biggest thing on my agenda was that I was going to give a 45 minute presentation to a group of patients and staff at 4:00 pm. Claire had gone shopping for another suitcase and a backpack and so I was on my own. Karen came with an IT guy around 9:00 am and we went to the conference room to make sure that all the systems were working so that the computer would display through the LCD panel on the wall. When everyone was sure that they understood how the systems worked we carried on with the PT, working on balancing exercises, and using fake weights to simulate loading luggage onto a luggage cart and putting carry-on bags into overhead compartments.

Having accomplished this task we worked on my balance on a variety of unstable surfaces, making me hold my balance unaided with my eyes shut, and then reaching to retrieve items from a frame in front of me, moving clips from a rack and setting them on a table, and then picking them up with my other hand and putting them back on the rack. This was easy until she asked me to use my right hand to replace items on my left side and vice versa. This was where I was really challenged.

After the balance exercises we did some more work with real suitcases since Claire had brought one to the unit that morning. My personal wheelchair arrived, so I signed the rental agreement, and paid the 20% co-pay on the rental, and Karen helped me set it up. I found it interesting that my co-pay for six months was more than the purchase price of a new wheelchair on the internet. After the wheelchair had been tested, Karen worked with me filling up the suitcase with even heavier weights, and after weighing it (it weighed 30 pounds) I then lifted it up onto the bed. Karen made a note on the white board that the physical therapist for Saturday should work with me on increasing the load and lifting two suitcases, as well as using a step stool, something I would need to use at home to fix things and get things out of high cupboards where I kept my important snacks.

During my next therapy session we continued on my work with the suitcase and she gave me some hints on how to bend my knees to avoid putting strain on my back, and ensured I knew how important it was to make sure that I never twisted my back. After completing loading the suitcase onto the bed, simulating the trunk of our Dodge Grand Caravan, we moved onto the wheelchair and practiced folding it up and loading it onto the bed, then removing it and putting the foot rests back on it. It weighed in at 31 pounds. After the late morning therapies, I had lunch in the dining area with the other patients, and after a perfunctory visit from Dr. Matthews, I retired discreetly to my room, where I had some time for myself, something that didn't happen a lot in hospitals.

Belinda Knowles, the woman who had come to visit us in the hospital to tell us about the rehabilitation unit, came by to see if she could take a video of me walking with my walker. She said she was going back to the hospital where I was initially diagnosed the following week and she wanted to show the staff there her star patient. I told her that I could walk without the walker, but she insisted that I use the walker since she didn't need me falling on the video, messing up my plans to fly home on Sunday night, and reflecting really badly on the rehab center. I walked around the dining room, and even picked up the walker to show how little I needed it, signed the photo/video release, and she told me that she was very satisfied with the final video product. I then made sure I was prepared for my 4:00 pm presentation.

Claire was back in time, and six people showed up for the talk; a 45 minute version of Claire's "Historic Award Winning Teamwork" presentation on the historic sail of USS Constitution in 1997 when Claire was the second in command of the ship. I stood up and presented for about 45 minutes, using only the back of the wheelchair for support. I had a lot of energy and the audience of therapists and patients got really excited about the story. After the presentation there was a question and answer session for which I casually sat down. In the space of a single day I had extended my presentation time from 10 minutes to 45 minutes and needless to say I was very pleased with myself.

Day 40

Claire had checked out of the hotel so we moved into what is called the Transitional Suite. It had a queen sized bed, a mini kitchen, a table and a chair. It wasn't really set up for an actual living experience, but it was designed to come a bit closer to a real home situation than the patient rooms. The idea was that you have an opportunity to be independent, and the staff was supposed to leave you alone, but of course they would be available if you needed something! We were looking forward to a bit of aloneness! I moved all of the suitcases etc. from the old room to the new room, and then practiced picking up suitcases and putting them on the bed.

Then we were scheduled for our last outing, going with Ciara, the recreational therapist, to the movies! I was given the complete assignment, looking up the times, planning the schedule, scheduling the taxi, and while the purpose was to check my cognitive ability in terms of managing my life and schedule, for me it would be more of a physical challenge to navigate in and out of the taxi and up and down the stairs in the theater, etc. We decided to take only the walker, not the wheelchair.

I called for the taxi and it was a Dodge Grand Caravan, just like ours, so it was great to see that I could manage putting the wheelchair in the back myself. We went into the theater, and climbed to the very back row, and enjoyed "The Expendables". In stark contrast to my usual practice I managed to stay awake during the whole show, but my choice of movie may have had the therapists concerned about my cognitive abilities.

After the movie we went to a Greek restaurant for lunch, and I enjoyed another welcome break from hospital food, after which we took a taxi back to the rehab center, and at shift change it was time to say goodbye to some of our friends in the rehab center. It was a mixed bag; I was happy to be going home, but I had made some terrific friends. Claire took a few photos of me with special people, and after dinner we watched a video together.

Now you might think that with going home the very next day, we would be able to end this story without any more complaints, but that was not to be the case. I was really tired, after all, I had had a massive day, and so Claire went to the nurses' station to see if she could spur them on in the delivery of my 9:00 pm medication. She told the charge nurse (not Hazel) that I was ready to go to bed and asked for my meds to be delivered to me in the transition suite as soon as possible, and she returned. We tried to stay awake, but finally gave it up, and went to sleep. At 10:00 pm there was a knock on the door and a nurse we didn't know entered. She didn't turn on the lights, but navigated across the floor using the light from the hallway, and she handed me a plastic cup and said "this is your chewable calcium" so I tossed the contents into my mouth only to discover very quickly that it was NOT my chewable calcium, but instead was my anti-seizure medication and it tasted AWFUL. Of course, the next cup she handed me she said was my anti-seizure medication, but of course it was the chewable calcium. No harm, no foul. We went back to sleep quickly, looking forward to 8 hours of uninterrupted sleep.

That was not in the cards. At midnight a nurse came in, again, someone I had never seen before, and said that she needed to take my vital signs. Rather than trying to educate her that the transition suite was supposed to be independent living, I just lay there and let her do her thing, and immediately went back to sleep. Then at 12:20 am, she came back in again, this time to do a bladder scan, something I hadn't had done in days! After waking up I explained that I didn't need my bladder scanned, I needed to be left alone, and so she huffed off, throwing over her shoulder that she would document in my chart that I had "refused" the bladder scan. There were no more interruptions until six hours later (we actually had six hours of uninterrupted sleep), when we were awakened once again for two pills which I was supposed to have after my breakfast!

There is no question that fully training a new person requires time, and when a new staff person is only going to be there for one shift, it might seem as though the training time is a waste, but it doesn't matter. It's essential for good patient care that staff be fully trained, whether they are there for a shift or for life, and that training must be ongoing.

There was a method to the madness of the transition suite; its purpose was to allow patients to have the experience of independent living in a safe environment. Besides totally interrupting our sleep, the nurses' intrusions also degraded the quality of the intended experience, and the error with the medication was unconscionable. Fortunately, there was no harm, however I can imagine that there are medications, which if chewed when that was not their intended way of delivery, could create a serious problem. Makes you wonder!!! We were so ready to go home!

Day 41

GOING HOME DAY!

We were scheduled for a night flight, thinking that the airport would be less crowded, and the airplane itself might be less crowded, so we had the whole day to spend in the suite. I had a busy schedule of activities despite it being Sunday. I was most anxious for one of them which was going to be with a physical therapist with Yoga experience. I really felt like I needed some help with knowing what I would be able to continue doing with the Yoga program on the Wii when I got home.

We went down to the activity room and had breakfast with some of the other patients, and while we were there Miriam came by to say goodbye even though it was her day off. She brought us croissants from her favorite French bakery for our breakfast, and we were very grateful. We then went back and finished most of our packing, and I started writing thank you notes using the hospital's "Gold Star" system, where I could give a gold star to a staff person who was truly helpful. The problem was that there were so many!!! We were truly blessed by a very high quality of care, and with the exception of a few people (like the nurse from the previous night) they all deserved gold stars!

Our ability to "officially" recognize the terrific actions of the staff was not always easy. On our own, we tried to get thank you notes to everyone who made a difference in the quality of our care, but when we found out that there was a way to do it "officially", it was even better. Sadly, we hadn't documented all of the names, much less the first and last names, of all of the people we wanted to thank. It would have been great to have been given a stack of "gold star" cards on admission, so that we could fill them out as we went along, instead of on the last day.

As it was, I wrote more than 25 thank you notes and filled out more than 30 "gold star" cards to thank the people who had made my experience a more positive one. It was a terrific feeling.

Suddenly it was lunch time, so we went to the dining room and joined the other "guests" for lunch, after which we had a little sleep, and then at 3:00 Karen came in after her hike, and it was her turn to say goodbye. At 3:15 the long awaited Yoga PT came! Jessica took me down to the gym, and showed me some ways I could do what I wanted to do successfully and safely, and I learned my own limitations and how to work around them, so I was very happy! By the time I finished all my Gold Star recommendations, and we tried to get a copy of my medical records, it was nearly 5:00 pm, and time to finish up our packing, arrange for a cab, change our clothes, make one last trip to the bathroom, and leave!

We said our goodbyes to the other patients and nursing staff and then Irma and another nurse helped us take our suitcases and me in the wheelchair downstairs to catch a cab to the airport. It was good that it was a quiet Sunday evening and we made our way through the security checkpoint with no problems, even with our wheelchair.

The night flight is called the red eye; I am sure because your eyes are totally bloodshot the next day from a lack of sleep. Claire can never sleep on a night flight, although I actually manage to do pretty well, but in this case she didn't even put up a moment's fuss about taking the night flight; in fact, she was totally in agreement that it was the easiest way for us to travel. We scheduled our trip so that we were early enough that we could eat in a sit down restaurant and I could choose real food from a real menu, and it was great.

Our night flight was actually far easier than either Claire or I had expected. Our decision to fly at night was a good one, there were fewer people at the airport, and it was easier to deal with security. Being in a wheelchair I was permitted to board first. I wheeled the chair down the jetway and transferred to the walker but it was far too wide. I used the backs of the seats to help me as I made my way to my designated seat, only three rows back from the entry door, and immediately behind the emergency exit rows.

Claire and I took our seats. I had the aisle seat and she took the middle and we hoped no one would come to sit in the window seat. We were lucky, and when the flight took off, on time, that seat was still empty. It felt wonderful to be flying home again. We were free at last.

Chapter 10 - Back Home and the "New Normal"

The van service Claire had contracted with was waiting so Claire wheeled me to the van and then got the suitcases. The drive home was uneventful and as we arrived in front of our house we passed our neighbors, Will and Laura out for their morning walk. It was great to see them after such a long and eventful time away, and we thanked them profusely for all their help during our period away. I managed to get into the house with the walker and Will helped Claire with the suitcases. It was fantastic to be back in our own home again, and in the fridge there was a complete meal prepared by Laura, enough for two days of dinners, and we were very grateful.

There was a lot of mail to sort through, and one of the things that had arrived was my new blue walker which I was able to assemble sitting in a chair in the kitchen. Claire started unpacking while I sorted through the mail, and then finally the big test! I used my walker to get around the ground floor before attempting to venture upstairs; the rail was now securely fastened to the wall, so I found that I could get upstairs to the bedroom level without any problem and wouldn't need the bed our friends had set up in the living room. We were astounded at how quickly my recovery made all our plans obsolete. We reminded ourselves that just a few weeks prior we had believed I would be coming home in a wheelchair and would need a ramp and perhaps a stair lift to get upstairs. We had more reasons to rejoice than we could count.

The next challenge was to see how well I could do in our own fitness center. Before the attack I would run on the treadmill, ride the upright bike, and then go to the pool; I was what you could call a "try" athlete. Claire had talked me into wiping out my history of results on the Wii Fit and that was a good decision. It would have been too depressing to compare what I was able to do now, with what I had done when I was in the best shape of my life the day before the attack. The old normal was irrelevant now and I had to set new goals, besides Wendy can be so snippy if she feels she has been ignored, and she had been, for seven weeks. I tried the reclining bike but it was soon obvious that I could use the upright bike just as easily, because of its walk through design which meant I didn't have to lift my leg very high to get on it, so I rode about 4 miles my first day, and then I did some yoga and some strength and balance exercises. We realized that with the additional exercises I would be doing we would need even more time in the morning before we would be ready to be out and about, so we planned to avoid morning appointments for the foreseeable future!

During our first meeting with my neurologist, Dr. Winters, we brought him up to speed on our adventures in California, and he was most impressed by the extent and speed of my recovery. He also reassured us that in the event I had any kind of a relapse at the end of the steroid taper he would have no problem putting me right back on the steroids, which we found reassuring.

After our meeting with Dr. Winters I took the offending laptop in to the retail store where I had bought it, along with a four year service plan that was about to expire. I explained that the power supply was running too hot, and they duly sent it off to the service center (as it happens, the fan had ceased functioning, which was what had caused it to get so hot that it had burned me).

It was finally time for the long awaited reunion with the grandchildren. Claire was still being protective, so she had established that the two families could come separately, and the first visit was with our son's four children. It was great to see the looks on their faces as they saw me standing upright, and after big hugs all around we sat outside on our deck and chatted as the children ate popsicles. Our oldest grandson reminded us that we owed him and his brother a sleepover, and his 5 year old brother proudly announced that he had completed his first two days in school without a detention. Our oldest granddaughter gave us a thank you note for allowing them all to use the lake house we had rented for a vacation and then been unable to use, and her younger sister spent 20 minutes snuggling on my lap. It was a slice of heaven.

Our days passed by, fairly uneventfully. We hired someone to do some yard work, spent enjoyable hours relaxing by the pool, worked out in the fitness center, and even went in the hot tub. I managed to get into the hot tub with no problem, but found that the 104 degree water felt cold on my legs, and it was only when the water reached my chest that I could feel that it was warm. I also realized that we didn't need to heat the pool for me, since at 76 degrees the pool water felt warm, until of course I was in up to my chest.

We met with my general physician (remember him from chapter 1?). He had done his homework and was pretty well informed about transverse myelitis even though when I asked him how many patients with TM he had taken care of, he grinned and said "You are my first!" He checked me over and like all my other doctors was pretty impressed by the speed and extent of my recovery. He told me to be careful and watch where I was walking, to always wear shoes, and he asked Claire to make sure that she checked my feet every night to make sure I had not inadvertently hurt myself during the day. He ordered all my medical records from California including my MRI films, and promised to be available whenever I needed anything. It was very comforting!

I had mentioned on Facebook that I had made scones as part of my occupational therapy, and one of our church members commented back that I had never made scones for them, so we decided to make scones for coffee hour on my first Sunday back in church. That, plus the normal requirements of eating and drinking, necessitated a trip to the grocery store, and in the evening it was time for our daughter, her husband and four year old son to come over for their visit. It was so wonderful to see them all again; my grandson had made me a special card and Claire got some great photos of him sitting with me. After about 15 minutes our son arrived with his youngest daughter, the one who had sat in my lap and cuddled with me the day before, and the two guys worked together to do some of the jobs that I normally did, but was presently unable to, like cleaning up dead ants off the pool room floor, cleaning the dryer filter, spraying the wasps under the slide on the swing set, and moving my wheelchair down into the garage since it didn't look like we would be using it again.

On the following day our pastor came by early in the morning, full of admiration for my ability to walk with relative ease. Together we thanked God once more for his many blessings. We had plans for the day to drive up to the lake where we had rented a cabin with some friends for a week of vacation. We of course had cancelled on them, but they were there enjoying their holiday, so we decided to surprise them with a visit (all but the one who knew that we were coming) and when we walked down to the beach I was greeted with tears of joy and great emotion. They had been with us in frequent phone calls and numerous emails throughout the ordeal, and the two women, who were both nurses, had done an enormous amount of research for us, and had provided tons of information and advice. We spent a very pleasant afternoon sitting on the beach, and when I went swimming in the lake I was again surprised to feel that the lake water felt warm on my legs, but when Claire splashed me on the chest I realized it wasn't really that warm. I was (and still am) very curious why lake water at 80 degrees feels warm yet the hot tub, at 104 degrees feels cold. It helped me to understand Sally Franz's book title "Scrambled Leggs". I guessed that my sensors needed to be re-calibrated. I had to agree with my friend, the heating and air conditioning guru, who claims that there is no such thing as cold; it is merely an absence of heat!

One time while I was living in Montreal there was a real lack of heat. We had parked across the street from a restaurant, and in the space of the few moments it took to cross the street, my beard and hair had frozen solid with ice crystals, and by the time we were done with our meal, a bottle of wine in the trunk had frozen as well. Luckily we had more heat at the lake this year, so it was a very pleasant afternoon, sitting on the beach, chatting with friends and relaxing in freedom for the first time in a long time, and showing off the results of my rehabilitation. I managed to walk up and down the steps to the house even though there was no railing on either side, which was a huge accomplishment, and everyone was duly impressed by my performance.

The next day was baking day, and to shepherd my energy we decided to bake the scones for church in two stages. We mixed the dry ingredients for 12 batches of scones and then tidied up the kitchen before going down to the pool for the rest of the morning. After lunch I got ready for the first of many physical therapy appointments which were in the plan.

I was startled to be introduced to a Roman Catholic nun, Sister Rose Marie, a Physical therapist, dressed in full habit, wimple and running shoes. After my initial shock I quickly discovered that she was very competent, extremely knowledgeable and thorough, and she knew a lot about TM. I didn't know that any other therapist would have been as aware as she was of the dynamics of TM, and realized that once again, I was blessed.

She seemed delighted that I had such good mobility, though she did explain that I needed to be careful to avoid overtaxing my muscles because that would make my recovery more difficult. She also explained that there would be scar tissue from the lesions on my spinal column, which she would have to work on, and that she would spend a lot of time working on my small muscles to make sure that my large muscle movements were more coordinated. I was glad that she was going to do things that I couldn't do myself; I had been worried that the outpatient therapy would be too elementary for me.

She also suggested that I would benefit from access to a pool for water exercises, and when I told her that I had a pool at home, she said, "Yes, but that will only be good for another couple of weeks". Her assumption was that we had an outdoor pool, and with winter coming, it wouldn't be available to me for long. I said somewhat apologetically, "Well, actually we have an indoor pool at our house." She gave me a high five, and told me that there were a lot of exercises that I could do in the pool that would be very helpful.

After lunch, Claire and I baked the scones, and by the time we had finished we had made nearly 300 mini scones; we figured that was plenty, and might even mean some leftovers as well!

Each morning I woke up stronger than the day before; perhaps because of the steroids. I would look at myself in the mirror, sorry that I wasn't looking any more buff, but guessing that there must be different kinds of steroids and I wasn't getting the "get me buff – help me play baseball" kind. My research on TM had taught me that steroids don't always work for TM patients, but in my case they were clearly working well. I was pleasantly surprised that I could actually do some of the balance exercises on the Wii Fit, as well as the yoga and strength training exercises, and now had a new baseline so that I could chart my progress on a regular basis. The water exercises were also really beneficial to me, and I worked hard on things like scissor kicks to strengthen my hip flexors. One morning when I was exercising I overbalanced while doing a lunge. I didn't hurt myself when I fell backwards; it was an open area and we had rubber sponge flooring, but it was yet another reminder of how careful I had to be all the time.

The grandchildren and their parents were now regular visitors, and by their second visit they were able to stay longer and go swimming again. I noticed that I had to leave the pool frequently to make sure that I was compliant with the "No Pee in the Pool" rule, but fortunately it wasn't a problem; my control was getting better.

On our first Sunday back at church, our friends were amazed to see me standing up, walking and talking to them as if nothing was wrong. One friend accused me (jokingly of course) of making it all up so that I could get the extra attention! It was wonderful to be back in the loving arms of my church family once again. I stood both before and after church for about two hours each time, chatting with people and answering questions about what had happened to me as they all enjoyed the scones! It was a good test of my stamina and endurance which were growing daily.

As the days went by, I was getting better at balance exercises, and I managed to do 30 push-ups, my yoga and strength exercises and rode 8 miles on the upright bike, before we went to the pool. Other neighbors, Todd and Ann, brought dinner, and Claire drove me around like a chauffeur to PT, to church meetings, and to go shopping, but I was anxious to drive on my own, so I asked Dr. Lawrence about it, and he told me that if I was truly doing as well as I said I was, he saw no problem with me driving. The next day Claire gave me a driving test and approved me to drive, once I had proven to her that I could drive just as badly as I had before. I was finally really independent!

Sister Rose Marie continued to work on my small muscles to fine tune them and improve my walking style. I guess she didn't like my gait, but I didn't take offence. She explained to me how the body compensated for injury by shielding the weakest link, and this was what we needed to work on to avoid things like a permanent limp. Everything she said made sense and at the same time, as a spiritual person, she could also provide spiritual comfort, so it was a one stop shop.

I was gaining in strength, and on day 51 I managed 50 push-ups, rode 13 miles on the upright bike in 1 hour at level 2, and managed the single arm and leg raise for the first time. It encouraged me so the next day I used the treadmill for the first time, and walked uphill at a 4% incline at 3 mph. Sister Rose Marie continued to be impressed with my improvement, and gave me a laminated sheet with pool exercises, and also a balance cylinder to use at home. The balance cylinder was basically a solid foam cylinder about 8 inches in diameter and two feet long, which you put behind your back and balanced on as you raised your arms and legs like a bug upside down.

Each day I tried a little more, impatiently wanting to do it all, but I had to be careful not to overwork my muscles since I wouldn't be able to feel it. My biggest challenge was trying to regain the abdominal strength I had once had. It just didn't seem to be coming back, at least not as quickly as I thought it should.

When Claire's cousin came for a visit, we went to see Spamalot, which was hilarious, and we all really enjoyed it, and I was beginning to feel more "normal"; my activities were now including more outside the house, and I was managing it all quite well. At dinner with friends to celebrate Claire's cousin's visit our friends who hadn't seen me since our visit with them at the lake commented that I was walking with much more confidence than the previous week, which was encouraging. Claire and I thought that things were going well, but it was great to get that reinforced by others, especially since the next day Claire and I were heading back to the scene of the crime; back to California to teach three classes, each lasting three days.

The schedule was to teach one class, then have a four day break, teach a second class, have a two day break, then teach the third class. We were going to team teach all three classes so I wouldn't ever be on my own, and while I felt that it wasn't necessary, it made Claire feel much better to know that she would be right there with me the whole time. That night, however, I had uncontrollable spasms in my whole body lasting about 45 minutes. I had had a few intermittent spasms previously but we had to be on a bus at 4:30 in the morning, and I refused to consider going to the ER.

When I woke, I felt cold but I managed to get up and get dressed and drag myself to the 4:30 am bus feeling puny and nauseous. I slept most of the way on the bus, and then on the flight, and by the time we reached San Francisco, I was feeling much better. When we checked in at the hotel the front desk staff on duty were all amazed at the extent of my recovery, and I didn't seem to have any lingering ill effects from the morning, so we didn't worry. During the night, however, I had intermittent spasms again in my right leg and then Claire woke up and was certain that I had a high fever, so after ibuprofen and a rubdown with a cold wet towel we decided that the next

191

day we would buy a thermometer so that we could keep track of my temperature.

On day 58 I was back at work. We hadn't brought the wheelchair, just the walker, and while I didn't really need it walking to class, Claire thought that I might be tired by the end of the day, and she could always push me in it like a transport chair (something you can't do with the low bid walkers provided by your insurance company). We had a much smaller class than usual, only 8 students, but that had been deliberate on Silena's part, to make sure I could handle the load.

Claire taught all morning and my first session was in the afternoon. Several of the students remarked that I looked normal, and they didn't even seem to notice that I was teaching sitting down in a chair rather than standing and pacing around the room. I had kept them updated weekly during my time in the hospital and rehab, so they knew that I had experienced quite the recovery journey.

We got a thermometer while out that night for dinner, and in the middle of the night I woke up with a temperature of 101.4, so that confirmed Claire's suspicions that I had a fever. We found an urgent care clinic on the internet that was nearby and decided to go there when they opened at 7:00 am where I wasted 30 minutes filling out a completely detailed medical history only to discover afterwards that they didn't accept my GIC coverage, nor did they have any way for patients to pay their own bills, either with cash or a credit card (perplexing). After asking them to shred my personal information I checked my temperature and called Claire, told her my temperature was normal, and we agreed to go to the ER after work.

Silena told us that there would be a fire drill during class at 10:00 am, but that I was not required to go down the 10 flights of stairs during the drill. I wondered what would have happened in the event of a real fire, and Claire found out that I was to go to the stairwell and wait; the stairwell was rated to withstand a fire for four hours, and that was plenty of time to send someone to help me down the stairs. The reality was that in the event of a real fire I had no intention of waiting in any stairwell.

Once in Seattle I had been stuck in an elevator that had dropped to a point between the 29th and 28th floors of the hotel. I was on my own, and it took them 98 minutes to get me out. I can tell you, it was not the best way to spend an hour and a half, and I was not about to be left in a burning building for four hours waiting for someone to come get me.

After class Claire insisted on taking me to the ER where the doctor ordered blood tests, a urine test (which I could actually do this time) and a chest X ray, and the only problem that they could find was a slight infection of the urinary tract. The doctor gave me a prescription for an antibiotic and explained that the shakes I had been experiencing were called rigors, and were my body trying to warm itself up and give itself a fever. With that explanation we left, prescription in hand, and went to a 24 hour pharmacy and got the medication. Around midnight the fever came back, but luckily my temperature had returned to normal by morning, so I could get back to work. My big test was coming in October when I would have to teach a four day class on my own.

The entire three days of the class went splendidly, and now I was on the antibiotics, and even though I still had a fever, it was only at night, and was lower each night. That was a really good thing, because a family emergency pulled Claire away for five days, but she felt that I was doing so well teaching that I could manage without her and this was amazing, since she was normally the hardest person for me to convince that I was OK.

I had promised Claire I wouldn't overdo it, so while I did work out, I made sure I didn't do too much, and the first morning, after my shower, I went down to breakfast and found there were slim pickings because they had been slammed earlier and all the good food was gone. (Note to self: make sure you go earlier to breakfast on weekends in future.) I got out my new "Yoga for beginners" DVD, and thought "what a joke" since the poses would have been a challenge to the Mongolian contortionists in Cirque de Soleil. I decided to dutifully attempt each pose at least once, but I decided that I would give up if I got my left foot stuck behind my ear.

During my second night alone I continued to take my temperature, and the highest it got was 100.1, so gradually it appeared that I was getting better. I reported this to Claire the next morning on the phone, and she reminded me to call the hospital and find out about the results of the blood work that had been done in the ER to confirm that my antibiotic was the correct one. My UTI had been diagnosed on the night of September 16[th,] and the doctor told us that he would know within 48 hours if it was the correct antibiotic, and if it wasn't he would call us. It had been 84 hours and we hadn't received a phone call.

When I reached a doctor, he looked up the results of my test, and confirmed that I had a urinary tract infection, which is apparently is quite rare for a gentleman, but I assured him that I was no gentleman, and he seemed satisfied by that response. I did, however, let him know that I had recently been catheterized about a million times, although the last time had been some three weeks prior, and he asked me what medicine I was taking. When I told him Lovaquin, he told me that Lovaquin wouldn't work for the type of UTI that I had; I needed Amoxicillin, so he phoned a prescription to a local pharmacy, and after working out I made my way to the pharmacy.

Interestingly, when I went for my follow up visit with my neurologist back at home, he told me that Lovaquin shouldn't be taken with my anti-seizure medication, since it tended to make the anti-seizure mediation lose effectiveness. Hmmmmmmmm. I know the ER doctor had looked at my records and seen that I was on Trileptal, but I guess he didn't know about that little complication.

Two days later the doctor I spoke with who prescribed the correct antibiotic called Claire's cell phone because that was the number in my chart at the hospital. While he was on the phone she asked him about the practice of calling patients back when the results show that they are not on the correct medication. He admitted to her that it was a procedural issue, that it was a problem, and that they were, in fact, having a meeting about it the next week. She told him to feel free to use our example in the meeting to develop a procedure that would ensure that no patient fell through the cracks that way. I hope he did!

After a good night's sleep with no fever or shaking (I didn't know if it was the new antibiotic, but things were definitely moving in the right direction) I woke early, and sat up at the required 30 degree angle after taking my Fosamex. While waiting the requisite 30 minutes at this angle, I used the Fosamex blister packaging to do some sharp/dull sensitivity testing, and while using it on my back I discovered that the line between sharp and dull actually depended on whether it was on my chest or on my back. The line descended my body from just under my right armpit, diagonally across my chest to navel level on my left side, and then continued across my back from my navel level on my left side, down to my hip level on the right side. It was like a downward spiral. I thought that this was very interesting; in the hospital the doctors had only tested me from the front, never from the back.

After yoga, posture re-education, abdominal and core exercises for the spine, the bug and crunches as well as balance and bridge exercises, I went to the pool for aquatic exercises, and after lunch I went to a meeting at work to talk about the requirements for an education program in Europe and was pleased that it looked as though I was going to have the opportunity to take my teaching program on the road to Europe starting in 2011.

Back at the hotel I stopped by the front desk and asked the hotel staff where I could get a great hamburger in town. The staff, helpful as always, mentioned a place that had just been written up in the San Francisco Chronicle as having the best burgers in town, and it was "just down the road". A coworker joined me at the desk, and agreed to go there with me. It turned out that it was a really dreadful plan; the road was El Camino Real and the restaurant was practically in LA. The taxi fare was ridiculous and the driver told us that we risked getting stuck in rush hour traffic on the way back if we hung around to eat, so I asked him if there was a discount for a round trip and he agreed to switch off the meter while we got our burgers. It cost us $47 just to get there, $33 for two burgers, one order of onion rings and two shakes; we ate in the taxi on the way back and we each ended up paying $60 for the privilege. Funny we won't be doing that again, and Jay will never let me forget that it was my idea! For the record, my Hawaiian burger was fabulous, my onion rings were good and my mango shake was excellent.

I taught my three day course with no problems. While I had the ability to teach standing up, I had promised Claire that I would teach sitting down to safeguard my energy, and that way I could stand up and explain things using the easel board if I needed to. I got a huge compliment from Silena's boss who told me that he was so pleased that I was back doing the work that I loved, and that they had a good thing going, using me, they knew it was a win-win situation. They were not looking to hire anyone else.

The next day at noon Claire was back, and I was really pleased. Emergency handled, she was able to get an early morning flight and surprise me at lunch time! Everything was now better! My temperature was back to normal, and it appeared that the crisis was over.

I think I could keep writing this book for the next two years (that is the amount of time I might expect to get some degree of additional recovery) but I am now sure that the worst is over, so it is time to end this book. I am now almost completely normal again. My new normal is not the same as my old normal, but I can live with what I have. Most people can't tell that there is anything wrong with me.

I have made some adjustments: Greg told me that every time I got up I needed to get my land legs, and now I knew what he meant. I have to make a conscious effort to make sure I am completely in balance whenever I stand up, and that all the communication systems are working before I start walking. I don't know if I will always have to do these pre-walk checks, but it isn't a bad habit. I will take this over a wheelchair or a walker any day. I still have several months of physical therapy left to regain my core muscles strength, improve my balance, and enhance my walking. My temperature and pain sensors are still not behaving, but this too I can work around. I am off steroids, and as long as I don't have a relapse, I should be fine.
As far as I am concerned, God kept His part of the deal, and I am very grateful that He did. I guess I still have stuff that I need to

do, so now it is time to get on with it. I have learned a lot about what can happen to you when you least expect it, about not taking things for granted, and what is possible with the power of prayer and love, and I knew enough to thank God.

OK God, you taught me a valuable lesson, that you are in control, not me.
I know I had been fooling myself all these years, but now I truly understand.
I was paralyzed and 60% of my body didn't work right.
I accept that you are in charge, and I am very grateful that you restored my basic systems.
Thank you for letting my brain still work.
I am very happy that you enabled me to walk again.
Thank you for taking away the pain.
I am very happy that I have some basic bowel and bladder control and I will never take them for granted again.
Thank you God from the bottom of my heart, I will always be grateful.

The "new normal" is just fine! On day 2 when I was paralyzed, and Dr. Thomas told Claire that there was a 33% likelihood that I would get some recovery, 33% that I would get full recovery and 33% that I would get no recovery Claire asked herself what she needed to be happy. It wasn't much. All she wanted was for me to have bowel control and she would have been happy; anything more than that was an extra helping of grace. We have had many extra helpings of grace. There is every hope that I will fully recover, and certainly the expectation that I will gain even more than I have today, after all, we are still as of this writing just at four months since the initial attack in the airport in San Francisco on July 20th.

We believe that there is a lot that is great about our health care system, but we also believe that there should be a regular process to discuss how all patient care is managed, and it should be free from judgment, and allow for freedom of expression. Yes, the Joint Commission has rules for how things should be done, but there are ways to make suggestions for improvement that even the Joint Commission will approve, but if there isn't a process within a hospital for making those suggestions, and if there isn't an arena for discussing them, nothing will get any better. Hospital staff should examine everything they do and don't do, to find areas where they can do things differently in a way that benefits the patient.

As a final note, we saw far too many patients who were all alone through the entire week and only had visitors on the weekends. Perhaps those visitors, those family members had been aggressively involved in the treatment planning, the research, and in asking questions before we arrived, but it wasn't evident to us.

If there is one lesson that is the most important, this is it: You have to be actively involved in your own healthcare, and if you can't, ask someone else to be, hire someone else to be, or beg someone else to be. It is essential if you want the best healthcare that America has to offer.

TM doesn't kill you; I wasn't in danger of dying, although I may not have gained as much recovery as I did if I hadn't been my own best advocate and had Claire there supporting me. We will never know; I was, and she was. We believe that my treatment was better because we had, and used, all available resources to ensure I got the best care possible. We have received blessings galore.

Epilogue

According to the dictionary, a hospital is "a place where sick people get treatment." It is rather like a people service station, where a patient comes in for some kind of problem and the clever mechanics run a few tests and suggest ways (usually involving things that come in bottles or with needles or knives) to solve the problem. The derivation of the word is from the Latin word "hospes" which means "to take care of". Yet in America, hospitals are businesses, and whether profit or not-for-profit, they have to make money.

It troubles us that making money is a motive when people's lives are at stake. We wonder why we put so much effort (and expense) into saving someone's life through radical procedures, when they have been killing themselves through their choices of food, drink, drugs, driving style, cigarettes, etc? Why do we put so much emphasis on the treatment of illness rather than on the prevention of disease? Why do we allow the rich to have whatever medical treatment they want, but we make the poor do without? Why do we call traditional, homeopathic or Asian remedies, "alternative" medicine when they have been around, and worked, for thousands of years? Why is chemical medicine "mainstream"?

Why are we the only civilized nation on earth that does not provide health care to all of its citizens? Why, after hundreds of attempts and millions of dollars, have we been unable to effectively reform our healthcare system?

We certainly don't have the answers to any of these questions, but we do know that there is a lot that could be done to improve America's medical system.

Who is the customer?

We always assumed that the "customer" was the patient but never felt treated like a customer. In our recent experience in hospitals there were no placards advertising that any of these hospitals had just won the JD Powers award for excellent customer service. There were no placards imploring the staff to remember that "the patient is the reason we are here" or "the patient pays your salary" and there were no signs warning staff that "if we don't serve the customer well, someone else will!"

We did get a form with "Patients Rights and Responsibilities" but it didn't say the kinds of things that we were looking for, things like:

- We are here to help improve your medical condition
- We consider you a valuable member of our medical team
- Let us know if you have any specific needs that we should be aware of
- We welcome your public comments about our service on Facebook and Twitter
- We want your visit with us to be as pleasant as possible
- We will treat you with the respect, dignity and concern that we would expect if we were a patient in your care
- We will ensure that everyone who is attending to your needs is fully aware of your current medical condition
- We will organize our services to meet your needs wherever possible
- If you see anything that could be improved, please fill out one of our suggestion/feedback cards which will be reviewed by our Executive Team. You will get a personal response within 4 business days.

In point of fact, the patient may not be the customer. In many cases the patient is simply the recipient of the treatment, the consumer of the product (pharmaceutical) or the consumer of the service (nursing support). The real customer may be the insurance company who pays the bill for those who are insured. Additionally, there are thousands of people employed by insurance companies (government and private), hospitals, pharmacies and medical offices who depend on this work for their own livelihoods. It is an extremely expensive and highly complex system.

As an example of the complexity, I (Keith) was on a drug (Oxcarbazepine, the generic form of Trileptal) to control atonic seizures (irregular brain activity without the spasms so often associated with seizures) and it worked very well until our pharmacy changed suppliers. I took the new (supposedly equivalent) drug for three weeks and developed asthma. When I looked up the formula on the internet I found that the second product had the identical active ingredients as the first, but nowhere did the formula list any of the filler ingredients used to make the tablets, so I thought that I might be having an allergic reaction to one of the filler ingredients. I went back to the pharmacy and explained the problem, and asked the pharmacist to please reorder generic #1, but the pharmacist told me that he couldn't. He told me that the company which manufactured generic #1 was out of business. I had no choice, he said, but to use the new replacement, the one that caused asthma.

Naturally concerned we researched the drug on line, discovering, much to our surprise, that the pharmacist was incorrect. We found the manufacturer of generic #1 and they were still very much in business, so after checking with two other pharmacies, we found one that loved the idea of our insurance company's $600 every three months and would get the product I needed with no problem. So now we have a new preferred supplier, not just for that drug, but for all our prescription drugs. As a patient, you may be totally uneducated about the product that you are being given, but you have a right to expect that it will improve your medical situation, not make it worse, and that your concerns will be effectively addressed.

Looking back on this experience we know that we were extremely fortunate to have been in the right place, at the right time, with the right doctors, who made the right diagnosis, started the right treatment in the right facilities. As a result of the excellent health care that I received I am almost fully recovered today.

How much of that is luck, how much of that is faith, how much of that is the power of prayer, how much is the result of the treatment, how much is the result of the exercises, how much is the result of a positive attitude, how much of that is the result of hard work we will never know, but we believe in the power of prayer and we always had faith that there would be a positive outcome.

Perhaps you have a loved one in the hospital, or you may be a doctor or a nurse trying to make a difference in the life of a patient. Whoever you are, we admire you, respect you, and pray that you will be successful and have your own happy ending!

Keith and Claire

For more information about Transverse Myelitis, please visit www.myelitis.org.

You can reach Keith by email at Klaunch@aol.com, and you can reach Claire by email at cvblcdr@aol.com.

Appendix A – Summary of Lessons Learned for Health Care Professionals and Institutions

Efficiency
If there is a more efficient way of doing something that will allow you to have more time for hands-on patient care, then suggest it, implement it, and use it.

Communication
The patient should never be the last to know anything! Whenever possible keep the patient and family fully informed at all times, about tests, test results, plans, staff changes and orders.

Medication
Let patients know the potential side effects and interactions of the medications you are recommending.

Spinal taps and other procedures
Tell the patient before a procedure if there is something that will help them overcome the potential side effects of a procedure, so that they can do whatever it takes to have a good outcome.

Case managers
Hospital Case Managers are responsible for, among other things, discharge planning. They are extremely important to the patient and the patient's family, so they should be assigned when a patient is admitted, and remain with the patient as long as the patient is in the hospital.

Ordering food
When a patient checks in, the staff knows that they will need food. After the initial crisis has passed, make sure that your patients and their families know how to select and order food so that they can be as comfortable as possible.

Patient and family support
Be alert for signs that patients and their families need some emotional support, and be prepared to call for assistance.

Staying in touch
Provide access to portable computers and video teleconferencing so that patients can stay in touch with family and friends.

Coordination
Insurance companies, case managers, doctors and patients must be able to communicate 24 hours a day, seven days a week, and be able to make decisions and plans no matter what time of day or day of the week it is.

Families
Sometimes you have to take care of family members as well. Be prepared to do so, either with nursing staff or special assistants who are knowledgeable about the area and who can help.

Stuff
People, especially people from out of town, have "stuff". Have a place to safely store it.

Policies
If you make them, then use them.

Procedures

If you have a procedure that you tell your patients about, then follow it. If it doesn't make sense, then change it.

Give your patients as much high quality rest as possible

Sleep is an important part of the recovery process.
Within the bounds of ensuring patient health and safety, make every effort to ensure that patients get the maximum amount of rest possible.

Adherence to schedule

In so far as possible, if a schedule is agreed to, try to maintain it. If something is scheduled at an inconvenient time, then reschedule it!

Security

Some patients will have items in their possession that they will want kept secure. Provide a place for them to store those items safely.

Spiritual counselors

Not every patient may ask for a visit from a spiritual counselor, but if a patient does, please follow through and make sure that it happens.

Families count too

If a family member appears to be in need of assistance, please mobilize support for them. Volunteers, social workers, or counselors should be available to help out as needed.

Not every patient in a teaching hospital is there to be your guinea pig.

Doctors have to learn, but there comes a point at which your teaching should not impinge on a patient's healing.

Accuracy
Check and even double check a report before you sign it.

Planning
If a crisis demands an immediate response, then make one, but if something can be planned and scheduled, and the patient's well being can be served by doing so, then do it.

Test results
If a doctor orders a test for a patient, blood, urine, or any other kind, the doctor should be obligated to report the results to the patient unless there is an agreement with the patient to do otherwise.

Maximize every minute for recovery.
If a patient is undergoing a treatment that leaves "free time", ensure that there are other efforts being made during that "free time" to enhance recovery. Every minute in the hospital should be productive healing time for the patient.

Issuing medication
Ensure that every time you administer medication to patients that you verify the patient's identity, the medication and dosage being administered, that they match, and that the patient understands the purpose of the medication.

Introduce new staff to the patient
When any new staff person comes into the patient's room, ensure that they are either introduced, or introduce themselves to the patient.

Talk <u>with</u> the patient, not <u>about</u> the patient
When medical staff discusses a patient's care in the room, the conversation should always be conducted WITH the patient's participation.

Take the time for full disclosure
An informed patient is an empowered patient and an engaged patient.

Training
Training staff to manage a function requires that they both understand the function and that they are able to perform the function. That training must also include how to respond to all the possible negative events that may occur while performing that function.

Quality of supplies
All incidents occurring which reflect on the quality of supplies should be referred to a board for review, to determine whether a new supplier is required.

Let patients know the plan
As the plan for patient recovery and discharge is developed, let the patient and his/her family know what it is; even if it may change, keep them informed.

Common areas
Set up common areas for families and visitors, so that they can have access to things they might need to assist their loved ones, or to feel more comfortable themselves.

It is one system, complex, but singular
The medical system includes the hospitals, insurance companies (governmental or private), and the patient. It is the people, the systems, the policies and the bureaucracies, but everyone is responsible; it is everyone's job to see to it that the patient gets the best possible outcome.

The Supply system must be flexible as well as economical
Where possible, purchasing leverage should be used to save money, but the system must be prepared for the same level of flexibility in getting new products quickly as it is in executing new treatment plans in the emergency room.

The total cost must be examined
Each part of the system must justify and bear its own part of the cost, but the true cost belongs to the whole system, and that is the cost that must be reduced to make our health care system efficient and effective.

Room transfers should not occur after "bed time" unless it is an emergency
Patient rest is sometimes nearly as important as medicine and treatment. Unless it is an emergency, patients should not be transferred during what might normally be considered to be sleep time.

Encourage examination of how things are done
Regular examination of how things are done can lead to process improvements that can make a dramatic difference to the quality of patient care.

Have the right material in the right place at the right time
Whatever supplies, consumables, or materials you need, should be readily available. The same thing is true for patient consumables.

Training
All new personnel, whether from within the institution, or from an external agency, should be fully trained on unit practices and procedures before they become responsible for patient care.

Reward and recognition
Have a well documented and well recognized system for reward and recognition of staff, and make sure the patients and their families know about it and have access to the tools they need to use it.

Specific patient care issues should be well documented
If a patient is ambulatory and will come in contact with visitors, and there are things that the patient should not be given, put a note on their chair, on their cane, on their walker, or around their neck so that no one accidently jeopardizes their health by a well meaning action.

Staff should ensure patient dignity
Staff should ensure that no patient has any private areas of their body exposed to non medical personnel at any time, and if a patient will be allowed out of his/her room the staff should ensure that the patient is properly dressed.

Ensure patients can use the products they have been given
Shampoo bottles may have to be pre-opened, as may soaps, tissues, creams or other consumable supplies.

Check for drug interactions
When prescribing medication, review the patient's records to ensure that there are no complications from competing medications. While not all drug interactions are known, all effort should be made to ensure that no patient is ever prescribed a medication which has a known bad interaction with another medication being taken.

If a lab culture comes back positive, verify that the patient is already on the correct medication.
Whenever a lab culture is done to determine if there is bacteria present, it takes some time, often 48 hours. By that time the

patient is usually on some medication. If the culture is positive for bacteria, verify that the patient is on the correct medication, and if he/she is not, call the patient immediately and prescribe the correct medication.

Appendix B – Lessons Learned for Patients and their Advocates

Be your own advocate, and if you are unable to, ensure someone else is!
As a patient you are partially responsible for the quality of care you receive. Ask questions, research diagnoses, research treatments, and if you are unable to do so ask someone else to.

Feedback mechanisms
Provide feedback to the staff and hold them accountable for providing feedback to each other. Ask if they have reported the information and to whom, and ask what response they received. Keep information flowing through the chain.

Efficiency
If you see a more efficient way of doing something that will allow the staff to have more time for hands-on patient care, then suggest it, ask that they try it, and if it works to use it.

Communication
Ask to be kept fully informed at all times, about tests, test results, plans, staff changes and orders.

Medication
Find out about all medication you are being given: what it is, how much you are getting, what it is for, and what the potential side effects are.

Spinal taps and other procedures
Ask if there are any potential negative side effects following a procedure and if there is anything you can do to reduce these side effects.

Ordering food

When you check in to a hospital or to a new ward, ask for a menu immediately so that you can make your own choices. If it is close to meal time, ask that your choices be faxed to the kitchen.

Patient and family support

If you or a family member needs some kind of support ASK FOR IT! Ask to speak with a social worker, a volunteer, a local minister, or anyone else who might be able to help.

Case managers

Hospital Case Managers are responsible for, among other things, discharge planning. They are extremely important to you and your family, so ask to have one assigned when you are admitted, and ask that the case manager retain your case as long as you are in the hospital, even if you are transferred to another ward. If that is not possible, ask for a full copy of all the notes the case manager has and ensure that they are transferred to the new case manager.

What to take or send someone in the hospital?

Take your loved ones cards, puzzle books, magazines, books, TV Guides, and DVD's if they have their computers, portable DVD players if they don't, MP3 Players loaded with music and/or audio books and food!

Staying in touch

If you don't have your own computer, ask for one to be made available to you so that you can stay in touch with family and friends. If one is going to be made available to you, ask about security considerations.

Coordination
Insurance companies, case managers, doctors and patients must be able to communicate 24 hours a day, seven days a week, and be able to make decisions and plans no matter what time of day or day of the week it is. If you are able to, get the phone numbers you can use to reach people after hours and on weekends.

Families
Sometimes family members need help too. Ask the nursing staff to provide someone who is knowledgeable about the area to help.

Stuff
If you have "stuff" ask for a place to safely store it.

Policies
If you are told that there is a policy about something, hold the staff accountable to it. If it doesn't make sense, then ask them to change it.

Procedures
If you are told that there is a procedure hold the staff accountable for following it. If it doesn't make sense, then ask them to change it.

Sleep is an important part of the recovery process
While it is important to get everything you need for your own health and safety, proper rest is an important part of the recovery process, so every effort should be made to ensure that you get the maximum amount of rest possible. Ask your doctor about allowing your door to be closed, the lights to be turned off, the noise level reduced, and the checks to be as unobtrusive as possible. If they agree, get the doctor to sign an order to that

effect. If you don't want to be woken for visitors, ask for a "Do Not Disturb" sign to be put on your door.

Security
If you have something that you need kept secure, ask for a way to do it.

Spiritual counselors
If you would like a visit from a spiritual counselor, ask for it! Sometimes, on admission, you may be asked if you want anyone to know you are there, and you may say "no" in which case that becomes a permanent part of you patient file. If this changes, let the staff know!

Families count too
If a family member needs assistance, please ask for it! Ask for a volunteers, social worker, or counselor to be made available to help out as needed.

Even if it is a teaching hospital, you are not there to be a guinea pig
Doctors have to learn, but if you feel that your rights are being abused, tell them to stop until you can have a meeting to discuss your part in the process.

Planning
If it appears that routine demands are being handled as though they are crises, ask for a few minutes to talk about the plan.

Test results
If there has been a test ordered, ask when the results will be available, and then ask for the results.

Maximize every minute for recovery.
If you have "free time" ask if there is anything you can do to enhance your own recovery. Every minute in the hospital should be productive healing time, and you may be able to assist in your own healing.

Issuing medication
Ensure that every time you are given medication that the staff verifies your identity, the medication and dosage being administered, that they match, and that you understand the purpose of the medication. If there has been a new medication added, a dosage change, or a medication removed, ask why! Do not allow any new medication unless you get a valid reasonable explanation.

Know your staff
When any new staff person comes into your room, ask them who they are and what their role is in your care. Ask them if there is anything they need to know about your case and your current condition.

Ask the staff to talk with you, not about you
When medical staff are discussing your care in the room, ask that they talk about it with you so that you can participate in the conversation.

Graciousness is always appreciated by families
Ask if there is somewhere in the ward that your visitors can get coffee or snacks, and if not, where they can get something. If your health permits, ask if you can accompany them off the ward or unit to the cafeteria or snack bar.

Take the time for full disclosure
An informed patient is an empowered patient and an engaged patient, so ask for a full explanation of all test results, all diagnoses, all treatment plans, and all discharge plans.

Quality of supplies
All incidents occurring which reflect on the quality of supplies should be referred to the staff and you should ask for them to review their purchasing decisions. Ask for feedback on what is being done and what has been done to solve the problem.

Keep things normal
As much as possible, keep things as closely as possible to what is normal for you in your own environment. Ask if you can wear your own personal clothing. Ask for assistance (if you need it) in getting out of bed and into a chair, sit up as much as possible and walk and stand if you can. Ask for a shower, ask to have your hair washed, ask to brush your teeth, and ask for whatever else you need to feel as though you are as close to normal as possible.

Know the plan
As the plan for your recovery and discharge is developed, ask to know what it is; ask to have your family kept informed.

It is one system, complex, but singular
The medical system includes the hospitals, insurance companies (governmental or private), and the patient. It is the people, the systems, the policies and the bureaucracies, but everyone is responsible; it is everyone's job to see to it that you get the best possible outcome. Be a participant.

Your treatment includes not only medication but also other treatments and procedures that are a part of health management
When you are admitted or transferred, make sure that any procedures, processes, and treatments that you have on an ongoing basis are discussed and addressed.

Have the right materials in the right place at the right time
Whatever supplies, consumables, or materials you need, should be readily available. If you need something, ask for it.

Training
You may need some training on unit practices and procedures in order to get what you need when you need it, before it becomes an issue. If you have a requirement for something try to ask for it before it is needed, and find out how you can keep the supply chain working for you.

Reward and recognition
Ask what the system is for recognizing and rewarding the staff, and ask for the required forms/supplies in advance.

Demand your dignity
Demand that curtains be closed, that gowns be secured, and that at no time you have any private areas of your body exposed unnecessarily. Do not allow yourself to be out of your room, whether in a wheelchair, or with a walker or cane, unless you are appropriately dressed. Ask for two gowns instead of just one. The first one open in the back, but then another used as a robe to cover the opening in the back.

Ensure that you can use the products you have been given
Shampoo bottles may have to be pre-opened, as may soaps, tissues, or other consumable supplies. Ask for help when you need it.

If a doctor orders a lab culture get confirmation of the results.
Whenever a lab culture is done it takes some time, often 48
hours, and by that time you are usually on some medication.
Ask when the results should be available, then remember to ask
for them and verify that you are on the correct medication.

About the Authors:

Keith Launchbury and Claire Bloom have been married (to each other) for nearly 20 years. They have four children, five grandchildren (with number six on the way), and live in New Hampshire. They enjoy travel and have lived in six different countries. Keith is an active business educator and consultant, and Claire is a retired Navy Lieutenant Commander and is also a business educator. They can be reached at klaunch@aol.com and cvblcdr@aol.com.